New Developments in the Understanding and Treatment of Autoimmune Hemolytic Anemia

Editors

ALEXANDRA P. WOLANSKYJ-SPINNER
RONALD S. GO

HEMATOLOGY/ONCOLOGY CLINICS OF NORTH AMERICA

www.hemonc.theclinics.com

Consulting Editors
GEORGE P. CANELLOS
EDWARD J. BENZ Jr

April 2022 • Volume 36 • Number 2

ELSEVIER

1600 John F. Kennedy Boulevard • Suite 1800 • Philadelphia, Pennsylvania, 19103-2899

http://www.theclinics.com

HEMATOLOGY/ONCOLOGY CLINICS OF NORTH AMERICA Volume 36, Number 2
April 2022 ISSN 0889-8588, ISBN 13: 978-0-323-98703-5

Editor: Stacy Eastman
Developmental Editor: Ann Gielou M. Posedio

Hematology/Oncology Clinics (ISSN 0889-8588) is published bimonthly by Elsevier Inc., 360 Park Avenue South, New York, NY 10010-1710. Months of issue are February, April, June, August, October, and December. Business and Editorial Offices: 1600 John F. Kennedy Blvd., Ste. 1800, Philadelphia, PA 19103–2899. Customer Service Office: 3251 Riverport Lane, Maryland Heights, MO 63043. Periodicals postage paid at New York, NY and at additional mailing offices. Subscription prices are $470.00 per year (domestic individuals), $1190.00 per year (domestic institutions), $100.00 per year (domestic students/residents), $495.00 per year (Canadian individuals), $100.00 per year (Canadian students/residents), $1232.00 per year (Canadian institutions) $563.00 per year (international individuals), $1232.00 per year (international institutions), and $255.00 per year (international students/residents). International air speed delivery is included in all *Clinics* subscription prices. All prices are subject to change without notice. **POSTMASTER:** Send address changes to *Hematology/Oncology Clinics of North America*, Elsevier Health Sciences Division, Subscription Customer Service, 3251 Riverport Lane, Maryland Heights, MO 63043. Customer Service (orders, claims, online, change of address): Elsevier Health Sciences Division, Subscription **Customer Service, 3251 Riverport Lane, Maryland Heights, MO 63043. Tel: 1-800-654-2452 (U.S. and Canada); 314-447-8871 (outside U.S. and Canada). Fax: 314-447-8029. E-mail: journalscustomerservice-usa@elsevier.com (for print support); journalsonlinesupport-usa@elsevier.com (for online support).**

Reprints. For copies of 100 or more, of articles in this publication, please contact the Commercial Reprints Department, Elsevier Inc., 360 Park Avenue South, New York, New York 10010-1710; Tel.: 212-633-3874, Fax: 212-633-3820, E-mail: reprints@elsevier.com.

Hematology/Oncology Clinics of North America is covered in *MEDLINE/PubMed (Index Medicus), EMBASE/ Excerpta Medica, and BIOSIS.*

Contributors

CONSULTING EDITORS

GEORGE P. CANELLOS, MD
William Rosenberg Professor of Medicine, Department of Medical Oncology, Dana-Farber Cancer Institute, Boston, Massachusetts, USA

EDWARD J. BENZ Jr, MD
Professor, Pediatrics, Richard and Susan Smith Professor, Medicine, Professor, Genetics, Harvard Medical School, President and CEO Emeritus, Office of the President, Dana-Farber Cancer Institute, Boston, Massachusetts, USA

EDITORS

ALEXANDRA P. WOLANSKYJ-SPINNER, MD
Professor of Medicine, Mayo Clinic College of Medicine and Science, Senior Associate Dean of Student Affairs, Mayo Clinic Alix School of Medicine, Department of Internal Medicine, Hematology Division, Core Consultative Hematology Group, Mayo Clinic, Rochester, Minnesota, USA

RONALD S. GO, MD
Associate Professor of Medicine, Mayo Clinic College of Medicine and Science, Department of Internal Medicine, Hematology Division, Chair, Core Consultative Hematology Group, Mayo Clinic, Rochester, Minnesota, USA

AUTHORS

ROBERT A. BRODSKY, MD
Professor of Medicine, Division of Hematology, Johns Hopkins School of Medicine, Baltimore, Maryland, USA

MAGGIE A. DIGUARDO, MD
Senior Associate Consultant, Transfusion Medicine, Mayo Clinic, Rochester, Minnesota, USA

MORIE A. GERTZ, MD, MACP
Roland Seidler Junior Professor of the Art of Medicine, Consulting Hematologist, Mayo Clinic, Rochester, Minnesota, USA

RONALD S. GO, MD
Associate Professor of Medicine, Mayo Clinic College of Medicine and Science, Department of Internal Medicine, Hematology Division, Chair, Core Consultative Hematology Group, Mayo Clinic, Rochester, Minnesota, USA

STEVEN R. HWANG, MD
Division of Hematology, Department of Medicine, Division of Medical Oncology,
Department of Oncology, Mayo Clinic, Rochester, Minnesota, USA

EAPEN K. JACOB, MD
Consultant, Transfusion Medicine, Mayo Clinic, Rochester, Minnesota, USA

CHRISTINE LOMAS-FRANCIS, MSc, FIBMS
Technical Director, Immunohematology Laboratory, New York Blood Center Enterprises,
New York Blood Center, Long Island City, New York, USA

TRISTAN F.P. MCKNIGHT, MD
Fellow, Transfusion Medicine, Mayo Clinic, Rochester, Minnesota, USA

MARC MICHEL, MD, MsC
Department of Internal Medicine, National Referral Center for Adult Immune Cytopenias
Henri Mondor University Hospital, Service de Medecine Interne, CHU Hopital
Henri-Mondor, Assistance Publique Hôpitaux de Paris, Université Paris-Est Créteil,
Creteil Cedex, France

LESLIE PADRNOS, MD
Division of Hematology and Medical Oncology, Mayo Clinic, Phoenix, Arizona, USA

KAREN RODBERG, MBA, MT(ASCP)SBB
Director, Immunohematology Reference Labs, Northern and Southern California,
American Red Cross, Pomona, California, USA

ANTOINE N. SALIBA, MD
Division of Hematology, Department of Medicine, Division of Medical Oncology,
Department of Oncology, Mayo Clinic, Rochester, Minnesota, USA

CALEB J. SCHECKEL, DO
Division of Hematology, Department of Medicine, Mayo Clinic, Rochester, Minnesota,
USA

SURBHI SHAH, MBBS
Division of Hematology and Medical Oncology, Mayo Clinic, Phoenix, Arizona, USA

CONNIE M. WESTHOFF, SBB, PhD
Executive Scientific Director, Immunohematology and Genomics Laboratory, New York
Blood Center Enterprises, Long Island City, New York, USA

ALEXANDRA P. WOLANSKYJ-SPINNER, MD
Professor of Medicine, Mayo Clinic College of Medicine and Science, Senior Associate
Dean of Student Affairs, Mayo Clinic Alix School of Medicine, Department of Internal
Medicine, Hematology Division, Core Consultative Hematology Group, Mayo Clinic,
Rochester, Minnesota, USA

JENNIFER C. YUI, MD, MS
Assistant Professor of Medicine, Division of Hematology, Department of Medicine, Johns
Hopkins School of Medicine, Baltimore, Maryland, USA

Contents

Autoimmune hemolytic anemia (AIHA) is caused by the production of "warm-" or "cold-" reactive autoantibodies directed against RBC antigens that may be of undefined specificity, reacting with all RBCs tested or may have an apparent specificity. Autoantibodies may be of IgG, IgM, or rarely IgA isotypes and their production can be triggered by disease, viral infection, or drugs; from breakdown in immune system tolerance to self-antigens; or from exposure to foreign antigens that induce antibodies that cross-react with self-RBC antigens. Increasingly, AIHA is being reported in patients following allogeneic hematopoietic stem cell transplantation and treatment with anti-cancer checkpoint inhibitors. Autoantibodies, whatever their etiology, interfere with pretransfusion testing of patients requiring RBCs transfusion making compatibility testing complex and labor-intensive. The availability of extended antigen typing by DNA-based assay has made transfusion of RBCs that are selected based on the patient's extended phenotype (e.g., D, C, E, e, K, Jk^a, Jk^b, Fy^a, Fy^b, S and s) a feasible option and this can provide a significant measure of safety as they avoid the patient being immunized to antigens absent from their RBCs.

Careful consideration of the clinical history with traditional testing such as an antibody screen and direct antiglobulin test (DAT) allow for the categorization of most forms of autoimmune hemolytic anemia. Based on the initial findings, specialized testing can further categorize disease entities and increase the sensitivity of testing. In this section, we explain the diagnostic findings of both traditional and novel testing and how their appropriate interpretations help distinguish the forms of autoimmune hemolytic anemia (AIHA).

Hematologists often rely on the results of a positive direct antiglobulin test to confirm a diagnosis of autoimmune hemolytic anemia, but immune hemolytic anemia can occur when no immunoglobulin is detectable by routine methods. Negative DATs in these patients may be due to a small quantity of IgG on their red blood cells (RBCs) (below detectable levels), or when low-affinity anti-IgG is present, or when the autoantibodies are IgA or IgM in nature. A panel of tests developed to detect immunoglobulins on these patients' RBCs may be performed in a few specialized laboratories. These tests can be helpful in instances whereby the clinical picture of AIHA seems obvious, but the laboratory values are misleading.

The causes of hemolytic anemia are numerous and a systematic approach is critical for proper identification and classification. The direct antiglobulin test can establish the diagnosis and subclassify the majority of autoimmune hemolytic anemias. Further testing to identify the driver of AIHA can have significant implications in overall management. Advanced testing for rare nonimmune acquired hemolytic anemias or hereditary hemolytic anemias may be necessary if DAT testing is negative.

Warm autoimmune hemolytic anemia (wAIHA) is an uncommon and heterogeneous disorder caused by autoantibodies to RBC antigens. Initial evaluation should involve the DAT, with wAIHA typically IgG positive with or without C3 positivity, and a search for underlying conditions associated with secondary wAIHA, which comprise 50% of cases. First-line therapy involves glucocorticoids, increasingly with rituximab, though a chronic relapsing course is typical. While splenectomy and a number of immunosuppressive therapies have been used in the setting of relapsed and refractory disease, the optimal choice and sequence of therapies is unknown, and clinical trials should be offered when available. Newer investigational targets include spleen tyrosine kinase inhibitors, monoclonal antibodies targeting CD38, Bruton's tyrosine kinase inhibitors, complement inhibitors, and antibodies against neonatal Fc receptors.

Cold agglutinin disease represents a form of immune-mediated hemolytic anemia whereby an IgM protein either monoclonal or polyclonal deposits complement on the surface of the red blood cell. Once complement is deposited, the 3rd component of complement is recognized by receptors in the mononuclear phagocyte system resulting in spherocytic extravascular hemolysis. This results in a Coombs positive hemolytic anemia with the peripheral blood film showing agglutination. In many instances, the source is a clonal population of lymphoplasmacytic cells in the bone marrow producing a monoclonal IgM protein. Traditional and emerging therapies directed against the production of the IgM may have a positive effect on hemolytic anemia. Success in the management of cold agglutinin disease with rituximab, fludarabine, bortezomib, and bendamustine has all been reported. Recent studies have demonstrated that the blockade of complement with sutimlimab can stop the hemolysis without the use of systemic chemotherapy.

Surbhi Shah and Leslie Padrnos

Autoimmune hemolytic anemia (AHIA) is the group of acquired autoimmune conditions resulting from the development of autologous antibodies directed against autologous red blood cell antigens resulting in red cell lysis. Beyond the presence, severity, and duration of hemolysis which can lead to symptomatic anemia, additional complications at presentation and during treatment require a high degree of clinical vigilance. These include among others cutaneous, thrombotic, renal disorders, and infectious disorders. Complications can be due to the presence of the pathologic antibody itself, the process of hemolysis, or attributed to treatment. Comprehensive management of AIHA requires awareness and assessment of complications at diagnosis, during, and following treatment.

Steven R. Hwang, Antoine N. Saliba, and Alexandra P. Wolanskyj-Spinner

Over the past decade, the role of immunotherapy treatment in cancer has expanded; specifically, indications for immune checkpoint inhibitors (ICI) have multiplied and are used as first-line therapy. ICIs include cytotoxic T-lymphocyte-associated protein 4 and programmed cell death protein 1 inhibitors, as monotherapies or in combination. Autoimmune hemolytic anemia (AIHA) has emerged as a rare yet serious immune-related adverse event in ICI use. This review describes diagnosis and management of immunotherapy related AIHA (ir-AIHA) including an algorithmic approach based on severity of anemia. Suggested mechanisms are discussed, guidance on ICI resumption provided and prognosis reviewed including risk of recurrence.

Marc Michel

Evans syndrome (ES) is a rare immune disorder defined as the simultaneous or sequential occurrence in a single patient of immune thrombocytopenia (ITP) and warm autoimmune hemolytic anemia (wAIHA) ± autoimmune neutropenia (AIN). ES represents approximately 5% to 10% of all wAIHA and 2%-5% of all ITP cases in adults and its mortality rate is high. When ITP and wAIHA occurred concomitantly, other differential diagnoses must be ruled out. ES can be primary or secondary and isolated or associated with another underlying disorder and secondary ES. The management of ES is mostly empirical with a low level of evidence. This review reports some new insights on this rare disease and provides some practical tools for the diagnosis and management of adult ES.

HEMATOLOGY/ONCOLOGY CLINICS OF NORTH AMERICA

SERIES OF RELATED INTEREST

Surgical Oncology Clinics of North America
https://www.surgonc.theclinics.com/

THE CLINICS ARE AVAILABLE ONLINE!
Access your subscription at:
www.theclinics.com

Preface

Autoimmune Hemolytic Anemia: An Old Disease with New Twists

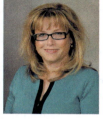
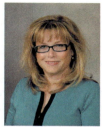

Alexandra P. Wolanskyj-Spinner, MD   Ronald S. Go, MD
Editors

In 1529, Actuarius in Constantinople was the first to describe "azure and livid" as well as black urine in patients exposed to cold. In his writings, he goes on to state that they also experienced a "dramatic loss of strength," likely depicting the first description of paroxysmal cold hemoglobinuria. Further elucidation of autoimmune hemolytic anemia (AIHA) would have to wait until the mid-nineteenth century when the observation of microcytes in the form of spheres (microcythemia) was documented in patients with non-liver-associated jaundice. At the turn of the twentieth century, the work of Drs Donath and Landsteiner in red cell antigens with the simultaneous discoveries made by Dr George Hayem, a prominent French hematologist, paved the way for the first description of an acquired hemolytic anemia. AIHA as an entity would require additional laboratory-based discoveries in the mid-1900s. It is therefore fitting to consider novel concepts and updates in a hematologic disease that is centuries old.[1,2]

In this *Hematology/Oncology Clinics of North America* issue titled, "New Developments in the Understanding and Treatment of Autoimmune Hemolytic Anemia," we review laboratory dimensions of AIHA starting with red cell antigen and antibodies from the red cross team, followed by a section on traditional and novel tests through the lens of transfusion medicine, and the evaluation of DAT-negative AIHA, from experts at the blood center of New York. We then turn to clinical dimensions, with an overview of the diagnosis and differential diagnosis of AIHA, followed by updates on the management of Warm AIHA and Cold AIHA, and complications associated with AIHA due to the disease and associated therapies. Our last section describes known association with AIHA, including drug-induced and immunotherapy-associated AIHA, and finally, the frequent clinical association of adult Evans syndrome. We are extremely grateful for the thoughtful contributions of these experts in AIHA and associated fields of transfusion and laboratory medicine.

Hematol Oncol Clin N Am 36 (2022) ix–x
https://doi.org/10.1016/j.hoc.2022.02.011
0889-8588/22/© 2022 Published by Elsevier Inc.

We would like to thank Dr Benz, Editor-in-Chief, for extending to us the invitation to edit an issue dedicated to this important disorder within benign hematology. We would also like to express our gratitude to the outstanding staff of *Hematology/Oncology Clinics of North America* for their expertise and guidance. Finally, we are indebted to our families for their tireless support and encouragement.

We hope you will find this issue focused on the state-of-the-art understanding and management of AIHA of value in caring for patients with this disorder.

Alexandra P. Wolanskyj-Spinner, MD
Mayo Clinic Alix School of Medicine
Department of Internal Medicine
Hematology Division
Core Consultative Hematology Group
Mayo Clinic College of Medicine and Science
Mayo Clinic 200 1st Street SW
Rochester, MN 55905, USA

Ronald S. Go, MD
Department of Internal Medicine
Hematology Division
Chair Core Consultative Hematology Group
Mayo Clinic College of Medicine and Science
200 1st Street SW
Rochester, MN 55905, USA

E-mail addresses:
wolanskyj.alexandra@mayo.edu (A.P. Wolanskyj-Spinner)
go.ronald@mayo.edu (R.S. Go)

REFERENCES

1. Mack P, Freedman J. Autoimmune hemolytic anemia: a history. Transfus Med Rev 2000;14(3):223–33.
2. Freedman J. Autoimmune hemolysis: a journey through time. Transfus Med Hemother 2015;42(5):278–85.

Red Cell Antigens and Antibodies

Christine Lomas-Francis, MSc, FIBMS[a],*, Connie M. Westhoff, SBB, PhD[b]

KEYWORDS

- Autoimmune hemolytic anemia • Autoantibody specificity
- Cold-reactive autoantibodies • Warm-reactive autoantibodies
- Direct antiglobulin test (DAT) • Genotyping

KEY POINTS

- Genotyping is helpful to support auto versus alloantibody specificity and is recommended whenever an apparent autoantibody demonstrates unexpected selectivity for a specific blood group system.
- Genotyping of patients with autoimmune hemolytic anemia (AIHA) is helpful in guiding transfusion therapy by avoiding alloimmunization and potentially reducing delays in treatment.
- Reactivity to Rh/Band 3 complex is more commonly seen in warm AIHA as demonstrated by the absence of reactivity with Rhnull cells.
- Reactivity to I antigen is more commonly seen in cold AIHA as demonstrated by the absence of reactivity with cord cells.
- Interference in routine compatibility testing can be addressed by demonstrating compatibility using adsorbed plasma or using units "antigen matched for clinically significant antigens" replacing "least incompatible" terminology. Clinics Care Points

INTRODUCTION

Autoimmune hemolytic anemia (AIHA) is a heterogeneous condition that is characterized by shortened red blood cell (RBC) survival due to the presence of "warm-" or "cold-" reactive autoantibodies that bind to RBCs with or without complement activation. The severity of the anemia varies from mild to life-threatening. Multiple triggers can cause the production of antibodies that cross-react with self-RBC antigens, including disease, viral infection thought to be due to molecular mimicry between autoantigens and pathogens, or drugs; from breakdown in immune system tolerance

[a] Immunohematology Laboratory, New York Blood Center Enterprises, New York Blood Center, 45-01 Vernon Boulevard, Long Island City, NY 11101, USA; [b] Immunohematology and Genomics Laboratory, New York Blood Center Enterprises, 45-01 Vernon Boulevard, Long Island City, NY 11101, USA
* Corresponding author:
E-mail address: clomas-francis@nybc.org

Hematol Oncol Clin N Am 36 (2022) 283–291
https://doi.org/10.1016/j.hoc.2021.12.002
hemonc.theclinics.com

to self-antigens; or from exposure to foreign antigens. Autoantibodies are also often seen in patients who are making alloantibodies, and common in patients who are chronically transfused and become alloimmunized. Identification of the specificity of the causative alloantibody in the plasma of the patient who also demonstrates auto-antibody reactivity can be challenging. The target antigen is often not clear as autoantibodies are almost always panreactive (reactive with all test cells in laboratory testing) but can demonstrate relative specificity (weakly or non-reactive with cells lacking common antigens such I, or Rh), and target antigen expression can be depressed or masked on the patient's cells when autoantibody is present. Lastly, AIHA can be seen in specific clinical settings including pregnancy, transplantation, and treatment with cancer immunotherapy.

The direct antiglobulin test (DAT) is a key laboratory test that determines if RBCs were coated in vivo with immunoglobulin (Ig), complement or both, and is discussed in greater detail in this issue. Briefly, a positive DAT associated with anemia and hemolysis without other obvious cause is suggestive of AIHA but the final diagnosis is dependent on the clinical and laboratory findings and include hemoglobin and hematocrit values, reticulocyte count, bilirubin, haptoglobin, and LDH levels. The RBC autoantibodies may be of IgG or IgM isotypes, or less commonly of both IgG and IgM, or rarely of IgA isotypes, with or without the fixation of complement. Not all autoantibodies (or positive DAT results) detected are associated with hemolysis or anemia.

The DAT results and the temperature at which the autoantibodies bind optimally to RBCs assist with the determination of the type of AIHA. Warm autoimmune hemolytic anemia (WAIHA) is the most common type, accounting for 60% to 75% of cases, and autoantibodies generally react at temperatures $\geq 37°C$. Other types of AIHA include cold agglutinin disease (optimal reactivity less than 37°C), mixed-type AIHA (typified by cold agglutinins that react at or above 30°C), paroxysmal cold hemoglobinuria (PCH), and drug-induced hemolytic anemia. More information on the diagnosis and differentiation of AIHA can be found in this issue by Go and colleagues

APPARENT RED CELL BLOOD GROUP ANTIGEN SPECIFICITIES

In the vast majority of cases, patient plasma will react with all RBC samples tested, and a relative or apparent specificity is not found, or may not be able to be determined by the hospital laboratory without testing uncommon or rare cells lacking high prevalence antigens. This requires referring the sample to a regional reference laboratory, which may be helpful to guide the selection of blood in some situations if transfusion is required and the reactivity appears to have a possible blood group specificity.

Relative specificities, which are seen when testing the plasma, differ according to the type of AIHA. The most common specificity encountered among warm-reactive autoantibodies is to the Rh complex, as reflected by the observation that the antibodies react with all cells commonly tested, but do not react, or react only weakly, with Rh$_{null}$ (lack all Rh antigens) or D– – (lack RhCE antigens) cells. Rarely, some have apparent "mimicking" specificity for a single Rh antigen such as Rhe or RhD or RhC.[1] These autoantibodies are referred to as mimicking because they can be adsorbed (removed) from the plasma by red cells lacking the antigen. If associated with recent transfusion, these "autoantibodies" can represent the immune response in an individual with altered RH alleles, with the antibody cross-reactive with the patient's own red cells. Genotyping is helpful to support auto versus alloantibody specificity and is recommended whenever an apparent autoantibody demonstrates selectivity for a specific blood group system.

Specificities to antigens in other blood group systems have occasionally been reported (**Table 1**). The autologous nature of an antibody may not always be obvious if the target antigen expression is masked, or transiently suppressed when autoantibody is present. Some RBCs can escape antibody-mediated hemolysis through selective loss of the antigen being recognized by autoantibodies (or even alloantibodies). This interesting phenomenon has been observed with antigens in several blood group systems. Antigen suppression has most often been observed with Kell blood group antigens, especially Kp[b].[2] Vengelen-Tyler et al.[3] reported a patient with a long history of idiopathic thrombocytopenic purpura who developed a potent antibody against a high-prevalence Kell antigen. His RBCs had profound depression of Kell antigens, but not of antigens of other blood groups. Transfusion of incompatible blood was well tolerated perhaps because the transfused red cells also showed acquired loss of Kell antigens. When the Kell-related antibody disappeared, Kell antigens reappeared on his RBCs and serum stored from the initial investigation now reacted with his freshly collected RBCs. Antigen loss or reduced expression has also been reported with Rh, Kidd, Duffy, Lutheran, LW, Colton, Gerbich, En[a], AnWj, and Sc1 antigens,[1] but it is important to rule out that the antigen is not detected (masked) due to interference from Ig coating the cells. If antigen suppression occurs, the patient's RBCs may test negative in the DAT although circulating autoantibody is present.

AIHA, after viral infection or vaccination occurs much more often in children than in adults. The most common autoantibody specificity is to I or IH. Very rarely, the autoantibody associated with infection may demonstrate blood group specificity. Giovannetti and colleagues[4] reported the case of a 5-year-old child with severe WAIHA due to complement-binding autoanti-Jka that was associated with Parvovirus B19 infection.

Table 1
RBC antigenic specificities reported in AIHA, characteristics of the DAT and autoantibody

AIHA Category	Autoantibody Specificity	DAT	Autoantibody
Warm autoimmune hemolytic anemia (WAIHA)	Rh complex, single Rh antigens (eg, e, E, C, Ce, c, D) Band 3 Also: Wr[b], En[a], S, LW, U, Ge, Sc1, K, Kp[b], Ku, Jk[a], Jk[b], Fy[a], AnWj, P[k], Vel	IgG or IgG + C3 or C3	IgG - binds optimally at 37°C; ~35% bind RBCs at 20°C
Cold agglutinin disease (CAD)	I/i Also: Pr, M, P	C3	IgM - binds optimally below 37°C
Paroxysmal cold hemoglobinuria (PCH) Donath–Landsteiner test positive	P Rarely: I, i, Pr, p	C3 Rarely IgG detected by special methods	IgG complement-binding biphasic hemolysin Binds to RBCs at low temperatures; hemolysis occurs at ~37°C
Mixed AIHA	IgM against I/i IgG panreactive	IgG + C3 or C3	IgG reactive by IAT at 37°C IgM agglutinating at ~30°C

Abbreviations: AIHA, autoimmune hemolytic anemia; DAT, direct antiglobulin test; IAT, indirect antiglobulin test.

SPECIFICITIES ASSOCIATED WITH COLD-REACTIVE AUTOANTIBODIES
Cold Agglutinin Disease

Cold agglutinin disease (CAD) accounts for 10% to 15% of AIHA cases. It is associated with autoantibodies that can directly agglutinate saline suspended RBCs at low temperatures (maximally at 0°C to 5°C); the agglutination can be reversed with warming. The DAT result is positive with anti-complement only as RBC-bound antibodies dissociate from RBCs at 37°C. Blood samples from patients with CAD, if not collected and maintained at 37°C until the plasma/serum is separated from the RBCs, often demonstrate spontaneous agglutination (the cold-reactive autoantibody agglutinates the autologous RBCs in vitro). This can cause problems with ABO/RhD determination and typing for other antigens.

The specificity of most cold-reactive autoagglutinins is anti-I; less commonly the specificity is anti-i. The I antigen is strongly expressed on all RBCs from adults (except on RBCs of the rare adult i phenotype) but not on RBCs from cord samples, whereas the reverse applies to i antigen. Autoanti-I is found in the plasma of most healthy people but rarely have a titer above 64 at 4°C. In contrast, the potent autoanti-I (titers are 1000 or higher) implicated in CAD and found in patients with lymphomas or chronic lymphocytic leukemia are mostly monoclonal (IgM, rarely IgG), with a broader thermal amplitude reacting at temperatures up to 30°C. Transient polyclonal or oligoclonal anti-I may result from infection, in particular by *Mycoplasma pneumoniae*. Anti-i, found much less often, is most associated with infectious mononucleosis and with immunodeficiency. Autoanti-i may be IgM, IgM plus IgG or IgG only. Rarely, specificities detecting epitopes on glycophorin A (GPA) such as anti-Pr or anti-M are seen in CAD, and further described in the section later in discussion.

Paroxysmal Cold Hemoglobinuria

Paroxysmal cold hemoglobinuria (PCH) is a rare form of AIHA and occurs secondary to a viral infection, especially in young children. With the increasing rise in the number of cases of syphilis in recent years (see Centers for Disease Control and Prevention) it should be remembered that historically PCH was associated with this disease.

PCH is caused by a cold-reactive complement-binding IgG antibody with specificity for the P antigen, an antigen expressed on the RBCs of all people except those with the rare p phenotype. The antibody, often referred to as a biphasic hemolysin, binds to RBCs at low temperatures but hemolysis does not occur until the complement-coated RBCs are warmed to 37°C. The antibody rarely reacts above 4°C and does not impede pretransfusion testing. In most cases, transfusion is not required but when it is, patients respond well to "random" RBC units; rarely have p phenotype RBCs been required. P antigen is expressed on many other cell types and tissues, including skin fibroblasts. The occurrence of cold urticaria in PCH may be related to the presence of P on skin fibroblasts. The standard diagnostic test for PCH is the Donath–Landsteiner test.[5]

Antibodies to Glycophorin Molecules

The most abundant cold autoantibody specificities after anti-I and anti-i are anti-Pr. These antibodies detect the protease-sensitive determinants on O-linked sialoglycoproteins that are predominantly found on GPA and GPB. Anti-Pr are IgM antibodies and are difficult to distinguish from (auto) anti-En[a] or (auto) anti-Wr[b] specificities but the distinction is mostly only of academic value as blood that lacks these antigens is almost impossible to acquire. Wr[b] antigen is located on band 3, the molecule that carries the Diego antigens, and not on GPA. However, Wr^b expression is dependent on the interaction between GPA and Diego in the RBC membrane and Wr^b expression can be altered or suppressed by changes in GPA. Autoantibodies to band 3 and in particular to Wr^b are a common finding in AIHA.[6] This group of autoantibodies has all been shown to activate complement and been associated with acute intravascular hemolysis and fatal or life-threatening AIHA.[7] For some patients, the clinical effects were far more severe than would be predicted from the serologic characteristics of the antibodies. A novel antibody-mediated mechanism proposed by Brain and colleagues[8] suggests the hemolysis may be independent of the action of complement and macrophages. He proposes that antibodies to GPA may induce lipid bilayer exposure and cation permeability; in particular, the binding of the antibodies to cell surface sialoglycoproteins may increase membrane phosphatidylethanolamine exposure and induce a Ca^{2+} leak.

TRANSFUSION CONSIDERATIONS IN AUTOIMMUNE HEMOLYTIC ANEMIA

Most patients with AIHA will require transfusion support with red cell products. The presence of warm- or cold-reactive autoantibodies can complicate pretransfusion testing and the safe selection of blood. As autoantibodies are directed against highly prevalent antigens, routine cross-matching is often unable to identify compatible RBC units. In the presence of autoantibodies, the failure to identify an underlying alloantibody may lead to a (hemolytic) transfusion reaction. Therefore, the aim of pretransfusion testing for patients with AIHA, just as it is for all patients who require transfusion, is to identify (clinically significant) underlying alloantibodies.

The extent of the interference will depend on the level of free antibody in the plasma, the phase of reactivity, and the potency of the autoantibody but also may cause problems with typing for ABO/Rh and other antigens. Studies of patients with warm autoantibodies have reported that the concurrent presence of alloantibodies ranged from 10% to 53% (reviewed by Zinman and colleagues[9]) or 12% to 40% (reviewed by Delaney and colleagues[10]). Underlying alloantibodies are a major hazard of transfusion for these patients, and methods to mitigate the interference of autoantibodies is labor-intensive and time-consuming as detailed in this issue by Jacob and colleagues The standard of practice for most transfusion laboratories is to perform either an auto or alloadsorption (or send to a reference laboratory) to remove the autoantibody and test for underlying alloantibodies at initial diagnosis. Transfusion of donor units antigen matched for more than ABO is an option that may eliminate the need for repeat patient workups if additional transfusion is required. This avoids the use of "least incompatible" units[11] and can be replaced with "compatible for extended blood group antigens." Transfusion of RBCs that are selected based on the patient's extended phenotype (eg, D, C, E, e, K, Jk^a, Jk^b, Fy^a, Fy^b, S, and s) can provide a significant measure of safety as they avoid the patient being immunized to antigens absent from their RBCs. The availability of extended antigen typing by DNA-based assay makes this a feasible option[12] (see later in discussion). The adoption of such an approach requires informed discussion between transfusion medicine staff and clinicians caring for patients with AIHA.

If an autoantibody has a clear-cut blood group specificity and the patient is actively hemolyzing, it is desirable to provide blood lacking the antigen as antigen-negative RBCs may survive longer than the autologous RBCs and may avoid an incompatible cross-match. In some cases that approach may come with the potential risk of exposing the patient to an antigen that they do not express, for example, providing blood negative for e antigen (which will be E+) when the patient lacks E antigen.

Generally, pretransfusion testing in the presence of cold autoantibodies is less labor-intensive as the antibody often does not react at 37°C and can be circumvented by performing testing at 37°C.

EXTENDED ANTIGEN TYPING BY DNA METHODS

No matter the approach used to remove the autoantibody to detect underlying alloantibodies, be it autoadsorption on the patient's own cells or alloadsorption (differential adsorption), discussed in detail in this issue, obtaining an extended antigen profile on the patient by DNA based typing is recommended.[12] A strongly positive DAT due to Ig coating the cells can interfere in antigen typing, most often associated with false-positive typing and/or spontaneous agglutination, but false-negative results due to antigen blocking can also occur. Removal of immunoglobin bound to the patient cells involves chemical treatment that is time-intensive and can weaken the expression of some antigens. A DNA-based approach offers more information at lower cost by testing for all common antigens in a single assay. The DNA blood group antigen profile also offers the opportunity to use this information to guide transfusion therapy with the potential to avoid exposure to antigens known to be highly immunogenic (K, RhC, RhE), or to transfuse the patient with red cells lacking common antigens that the patient also lacks, referred to as prophylactic antigen matching (PAM). Just as importantly, the extended antigen profile reveals what alloantibodies the patient may be at risk to make. This information can decrease the complexity of the laboratory workup, can reduce the number of repeat workups, and potentially avoid delay for subsequent transfusions and reduce costs.[12,13]

AUTOIMMUNE HEMOLYTIC ANEMIA ASSOCIATED WITH TRANSPLANTATION AND ANTICANCER DRUG THERAPY

There are an increasing number of reports of AIHA associated with transplantation and following treatment with anticancer drugs. AIHA can be particularly severe and life-threatening after allogeneic hematopoietic stem cell transplantation (HSCT)[14] and treatment with anticancer checkpoint inhibitors (CPIs), as described in this issue.[15]

Passenger lymphocyte syndrome (PLS) results when the donor lymphocytes passively transferred within the graft produce antibodies against the recipient RBCs. This generally can occur 3 to 24 days posttransplant and is usually mild and transient and primarily involves group O donors and ABO antibodies. However, antibodies to blood group antigens other than A and B associated with passenger lymphocytes have caused hemolytic anemia, including anti-Jk[a] following allogenic peripheral blood progenitor cell (PBPC) transplantation.[16] PLS has also been seen in patients transfused with allogeneic natural killer cells for the treatment of solid malignancies.[17]

AIHA after allogeneic HSCT has an incidence between 4% and 6%[14] and both warm and cold autoantibodies can be observed. Severe immune hemolysis is associated with high mortality and is challenging to treat due to concomitant factors including infection, graft failure, CMV reactivation, and GVHD. The DAT is almost always positive and may be positive for specific alloantibodies characteristic of delayed hemolytic transfusion reactions, or for donor-derived antibodies produced by passenger lymphocytes, and often accompanied by panreactive autoantibodies. AIHA in allo-HSCT is often reticent to standard therapies, although rituximab and several new options, including daratumumab, sirolimus, bortezomib, abatacept, and complement inhibitors are increasingly being used for this very serious complication.[18,19]

Antitumor immunotherapy, specifically CPIs that reactivate T lymphocytes to recognize cancer cells by blocking CTLA-4 or PD-1 are effective in numerous types of cancer. Potentially fatal AIHA has been reported.[15] Most cases were IgG positive warm AIHA; CADs were rarer. All were severe, with 80% of cases developing transfusion-dependent anemia, and the risk seemed higher with PD-1 or PD-L1. Mortality was as high as 17%.[15,20]

TRANSFUSION CONSIDERATIONS FOR AUTOIMMUNE HEMOLYTIC ANEMIA ASSOCIATED WITH PASSENGER LYMPHOCYTE SYNDROME, ALLOGENIC HEMATOPOIETIC STEM CELL TRANSPLANTATION, AND CHECKPOINT INHIBITORS

As in primary AIHA, the presence of autoantibodies directed against highly prevalent antigens interfere with routine cross-matching methods, and like primary AIHA, the challenge and concerns are to identify any underlying alloantibody specificities to transfuse RBCs lacking the antigen(s). Incompatibility associated with PLS and solid organ transplant is often transient and usually involves ABO antibodies, which can be addressed by transfusion with Group O donor units, or antigen-negative RBCs when the antibody is directed to other than A or B antigens.

However, with allo-HSCT, there is heightened concern and risk of underlying patient immune response to engrafting foreign donor red cell antigens, as well as risk that donor passenger lymphocytes are responding to recipient RBCs antigens. Transfusion management of post–allo-HSCT is complex and extended phenotyping is advisable to guide therapy to provide the best matched RBC units, as transfusion may lead to (additional) alloantibody production causing serious acute or delayed hemolytic transfusion reactions. A close collaboration between clinicians and the transfusion service is advisable for the best management of transfusion support in post–allo-HSCT.[21] Consideration for the best choice of red cells for transfusion therapy can be aided by the consideration of the pretransplant RBC extended phenotype of the patient and the extended phenotype of the transplant donor. If recipient pretransplant sample is not available, extended typing using buccal swab DNA should be performed.[12]

SUMMARY

AIHA is the result of the increased destruction of RBCs in the presence of anti-RBC autoantibodies and/or complement. Autoantibodies may be of undefined specificity, reacting with all RBCs tested or may have an apparent specificity. Those with a definable specificity have targeted RBC antigens in many blood group systems but Rh, Kell, I, and i predominate. Suppression of the target antigen concurrent with autoantibody formation may make it impossible to distinguish allo-from autoantibody by serologic tests (eg, anti-Kp^b, anti-e) and antigenic variation should be ruled out by genotyping. Increasingly, AIHA is being reported in patients following allogeneic HSCT and treatment with anticancer CPIs. Autoantibodies, whatever their etiology, interfere with the pretransfusion testing of patients requiring RBCs transfusion making compatibility testing complex and labor-intensive. Transfusion of RBCs that are selected based on the patient's extended phenotype (eg, D, C, E, e, K, Jk^a, Jk^b, Fy^a, Fy^b, S, and s) can provide a significant measure of safety as they avoid the patient being immunized to antigens absent from their RBCs. The availability of extended antigen typing by DNA-based assay has made this a feasible option.

CLINICS CARE POINT

- Pretransfusion and compatibility testing for patients with autoimmune hemolytic anemia (AIHA) is complicated and prolonged by the presence of warm-reactive autoantibodies that may mask underlying alloantibodies.

- Performing an extended blood group antigen profile and choosing donor units based on avoiding the stimulation of blood group alloantibodies can increase transfusion safety for patients with AIHA.

- If the plasma of a patient with AIHA demonstrates an antibody to a high prevalence antigen it is essential to determine if it is allo or autoantibody to avoid delay in finding blood for transfusion and to use rare resources appropriately.

- A positive result in the DAT is not an indication that the patient is actively hemolyzing.

- The Donath–Landsteiner test is diagnostic of paroxysmal cold hemoglobinuria (PCH)

CONFLICT OF INTEREST

The authors declare no competing interests.

REFERENCES

1. Garratty G, Petz LD. Immune hemolytic anemias. Philadelphia (PA): Churchill Livingstone; 2004.
2. Lee E, Burgess G, Win N. Autoimmune hemolytic anemia and a further example of autoanti-Kpb. Immunohematology 2005;21:119–21.
3. Vengelen-Tyler V, Gonzalez B, Garratty G, et al. Acquired loss of red cell Kell antigens. Br J Haematol 1987;65:231–4.
4. Giovannetti G, Pauselli S, Barrella G, et al. Severe warm autoimmune haemolytic anaemia due to anti-Jk(a) autoantibody associated with Parvovirus B19 infection in a child. Blood Transfus 2013;11:634–5.
5. AABB technical manual. 20th Edition. Bethesda, (MD): AABB; 2020.
6. Leddy JP, Falany JL, Kissel GE, et al. Erythrocyte membrane proteins reactive with human (warm-reacting) anti-red cell autoantibodies. J Clin Invest 1993;91:1672–80.
7. Nedelcu E, Desai M, Green J, et al. Acute autoimmune hemolytic anemia due to anti-En(a) autoantibody successfully treated with rituximab. Transfusion 2018;58:176–80.
8. Brain MC, Ruether B, Valentine K, et al. Life-threatening hemolytic anemia due to an autoanti-Pr cold agglutinin: evidence that glycophorin A antibodies may induce lipid bilayer exposure and cation permeability independent of agglutination. Transfusion 2010;50:292–301.
9. Ziman A, Cohn C, Carey PM, et al. the Biomedical Excellence for Safer Transfusion C. Warm-reactive (immunoglobulin G) autoantibodies and laboratory testing best practices: review of the literature and survey of current practice. Transfusion 2017;57:463–77.
10. Delaney M, Apelseth TO, Bonet Bub C, et al. Red-blood-cell alloimmunization and prophylactic antigen matching for transfusion in patients with warm autoantibodies. Vox Sang 2020;115:515–24.
11. Petz LD. "Least incompatible" units for transfusion in autoimmune hemolytic anemia: should we eliminate this meaningless term? A commentary for clinicians and transfusion medicine professionals. Transfusion 2003;43:1503–7.

12. Westhoff CM. Blood group genotyping. Blood 2019;133:1814–20.
13. Shirey RS, Boyd JS, Parwani AV, et al. Prophylactic antigen-matched donor blood for patients with warm autoantibodies: an algorithm for transfusion management. Transfusion 2002;42:1435–41.
14. Barcellini W, Fattizzo B, Zaninoni A. Management of refractory autoimmune hemolytic anemia after allogeneic hematopoietic stem cell transplantation: current perspectives. J Blood Med 2019;10:265–78.
15. Postow MA, Hellmann MD. Adverse Events Associated with Immune Checkpoint Blockade. N Engl J Med 2018;378:1165.
16. Leo A, Lenz V, Winteroll S. Nonhemolytic passenger lymphocyte syndrome with anti-Jk after allogeneic peripheral blood progenitor cell transplantation. Transfusion 2004;44:1259–60.
17. Skeate R, Singh C, Cooley S, et al. Hemolytic anemia due to passenger lymphocyte syndrome in solid malignancy patients treated with allogeneic natural killer cell products. Transfusion 2013;53:419–23.
18. Fattizzo B, Serpenti F, Giannotta JA, et al. Difficult Cases of Paroxysmal Nocturnal Hemoglobinuria: Diagnosis and Therapeutic Novelties. J Clin Med 2021;10.
19. Kruizinga MD, van Tol MJD, Bekker V, et al. Risk Factors, Treatment, and Immune Dysregulation in Autoimmune Cytopenia after Allogeneic Hematopoietic Stem Cell Transplantation in Pediatric Patients. Biol Blood Marrow Transplant 2018; 24:772–8.
20. Zhuang J, Du J, Guo X, et al. Clinical diagnosis and treatment recommendations for immune checkpoint inhibitor related hematological adverse events. Thorac Cancer 2020;11:799–804.
21. Barcellini W, Fattizzo B. The Changing Landscape of Autoimmune Hemolytic Anemia. Front Immunol 2020;11:946.

New Developments in the Understanding and Treatment of Autoimmune Hemolytic Anemia: Traditional and Novel Tests

Tristan F.P. McKnight, MD, Maggie A. DiGuardo, MD,
Eapen K. Jacob, MD*

KEYWORDS

- Autoimmune hemolytic anemia • AIHA • DAT-Positive

KEY POINTS

- Correlation of clinical history, standard laboratory, and transfusion laboratory testing is critical to properly diagnosing autoimmune hemolytic anemia (AIHA).
- The standard ABO type, antibody screen, and direct antiglobulin test (DAT) is a key starting point in the evaluation.
- Dialogue between the clinical provider and the laboratorian can help with test selection and interpretation of findings.

BACKGROUND

Autoimmune hemolytic anemias (AIHAs) are heterogeneous disorders characterized by antibody-mediated red blood cell destruction. The destruction of red blood cells may take place in the intravascular space if the immune response results in the activation of the classical complement cascade or, more commonly, in the extravascular space when macrophages in the spleen and liver phagocytose opsonized red cells. The risk for intravascular or extravascular hemolysis is determined by the presence or absence of complement and/or immunoglobulin on the red blood cells. This risk can be assessed by serologic investigations carried out in the transfusion medicine laboratory, which guides a more precise diagnostic workup essential to providing appropriate therapeutic management.

The monospecific direct antiglobulin test (DAT) is a standard laboratory test used to determine if a patient's red blood cells have been coated in vivo with immunoglobulin,

Division of Transfusion Medicine, Mayo Clinic, 200 First St SW, Rochester, MN 55905, USA
* Corresponding author.
E-mail address: Jacob.Eapen@mayo.edu

Hematol Oncol Clin N Am 36 (2022) 293–305
https://doi.org/10.1016/j.hoc.2021.11.003
0889-8588/22/© 2021 Elsevier Inc. All rights reserved.

hemonc.theclinics.com

complement, or both. However, the DAT result alone does not define AIHA. A positive DAT may or may not be associated with immune-mediated hemolysis, and as shown in **Box 1**, there are multiple causes for a positive DAT result that are unrelated to immune-mediated hemolysis. Therefore, clinical findings and additional laboratory data, such as hemoglobin or hematocrit values, bilirubin, haptoglobin and lactate dehydrogenase (LDH) levels, reticulocyte count, and red blood cell morphology must be considered in addition to the DAT result. Likewise, standard transfusion tests such as a type and screen, the DAT and eluate as well as more specialized testing found in reference laboratories such as adsorptions, the Donath–Landsteiner test, and the modified monocyte assay (MMA) may be beneficial in the diagnostic workup of AIHA when used and interpreted appropriately. Understanding the value and limitations of the available tests is critical to appropriate test utilization and interpretation.

DISCUSSION
Overview of Autoimmune Hemolytic Anemia Classification

At the most basic level, the AIHAs are classified as "warm," "cold," and "mixed" forms. Warm forms of AIHA are typically polyclonal IgG autoantibodies and optimally reactive with red blood cells at 37°C; however, IgM or IgA autoantibodies can also present. The DAT results in warm forms may be variable; whereas, some older data indicate that the DAT results are most commonly positive for both IgG and complement more recent data show that more warm autoimmune hemolytic anemia (WAIHA) cases are positive for IgG only (43%) than those positive for both IgG and complement (17%).[1,2] Cold forms of AIHA are due to IgM, which is typically reactive at 22°C or below and has an optimal temperature of reaction at 4°C. These are often directed against the I/i system. IgM fixes complement more efficiently than other antibody isotypes and thus is more prone to cause intravascular hemolysis. The amount of red blood cell destruction by intravascular hemolysis is understood to be 200 mL of RBC in 1 hour; whereas, the destruction by extravascular hemolysis is 10-fold less.[3]

Recent recommendations from the First International Consensus Meeting provided standardization to the definitions of AIHA, and the appropriate definitions are provided in **Table 1** for diseases discussed in this article. Regardless of the specific criteria, it is often the isotype and optimal reactivity temperature of the antibody that categorize the AIHA into either WAIHA, cold agglutinin syndrome (CAS) or cold agglutinin disease

---

Box 1
Causes of a positive dat[5]

Auto- or alloantibodies to red blood cell antigens

Drug-induced antibodies to red blood cell antigens

Passively acquired antibodies (eg, from IVIG, antilymphocyte or antithymocyte globulin, or donor platelets/plasma)

Nonspecific adsorbed proteins (eg, hypergammaglobulinemia)

Complement activation due to bacterial infections

Sickle cell disease, beta-thalassemia

Autoimmune disorders

Modified from: Borge PD, Mansfield PM. The Positive Direct Antiglobulin Test and Immune-Mediated Hemolysis. In: Cohn CS, Delaney M, Johnson ST, Katz LM, eds. Technical Manual. 20th ed. Bethesda, MD: AABB; 2020:429-478.

Table 1
Disease definitions in AIHA[6]

Autoimmune Hemolytic Anemia (AIHA)	Hemolytic Anemia Caused by Antibody-Mediated Destruction of RBCs.
Warm AIHA (WAIHA)	WAIHA characteristically has a DAT positive for IgG, IgA (rarely), or C3d ± IgG and a clinically significant cold reactive antibody has been excluded.
Cold agglutinin disease (CAD)	CAD typically has a DAT positive for complement (and negative or weakly positive with IgG) and a cold agglutinin (CA) titer of 64 or greater at 4°C. Patients may have a B-cell clonal lymphoproliferative disorder without clinical or radiological evidence of malignancy.
Cold agglutinin syndrome (CAS)	CAS often has a DAT positive for complement (and negative or weakly positive with IgG) and a CA titer of 64 or greater at 4°C. Patients have an associated condition such as autoimmune disorder, infection, B-cell lymphoma, or other malignancy.
Mixed AIHA	Mixed AIHA is diagnosed in patients with a DAT positive for both complement and IgG. There is a cold antibody with a thermal amplitude ≥30°C and evidence of a warm IgG antibody.
Paroxysmal cold hemoglobinuria (PCH)	PCH is diagnosed in patients with hemolysis and a positive Donath–Landsteiner test.

Modified from: Jager U, Barcellini W, Broome CM, et al. Diagnosis and treatment of autoimmune hemolytic anemia in adults: Recommendations from the First International Consensus Meeting. *Blood Rev.* 2020;41:100648.

(CAD), mixed-type AIHA, or paroxysmal cold hemoglobinuria (PCH). WAIHA is classically defined by DAT-positive for IgG with or without complement. CAS and CAD are both DAT-positive for the complement, typically have anti-I immunoglobulin specificity and have a cold agglutinin titer greater than 64. Differentiation of these 2 entities will be discussed later in discussion. Mixed-type AIHA has elements of both warm and cold forms; it is DAT-positive for complement and IgG and has evidence of both a cold antibody with a thermal amplitude at or greater than 30°C and a warm IgG antibody. PCH is a rare finding of a biphasic anti-P immunoglobulin that fixes complement at cold temperatures and then causes hemolysis at 37°C. PCH is diagnosed with the Donath–Landsteiner test, which is often only available at reference laboratories. The details of the Donath–Landsteiner test are discussed later in discussion. **Table 2** shows the typical serologic characteristics of the AIHAs.

STANDARD TESTING
Type and Screen

The start of any work up in transfusion medicine should begin with the blood group type and antibody screen. This provides valuable information including a basic forward and reverse typing, which defines the ABO type of the patient and demonstrates the presence of anti-A and anti-B in their plasma. The forward and reverse typing should correspond, or discrepancies investigated further. The antibody screen can hint at pan-reactive antibodies versus alloantibodies reactive with just one or more

Table 2
Types of AIHA[5,6]

	WAIHA	CAS/CAD	MIXED-TYPE AIHA	PCH
DAT (Routine)	IgG ± Complement	Complement only	IgG + Complement	Complement only
Ig Type	IgG	IgM	IgG, IgM	IgG
Eluate	IgG	Nonreactive	IgG	Nonreactive
Specificity	Pan-reactive	Usually anti-I/i	Usually unclear	Anti-P
In Vivo Hemolysis	Extravascular	Intravascular	Extravascular and Intravascular	Intravascular

Modified from: Borge PD, Mansfield PM. The Positive Direct Antiglobulin Test and Immune-Mediated Hemolysis. In: Cohn CS, Delaney M, Johnson ST, Katz LM, eds. *Technical Manual.* 20th ed. Bethesda, MD: AABB; 2020:429-478. Jager U, Barcellini W, Broome CM, et al. Diagnosis and treatment of autoimmune hemolytic anemia in adults: Recommendations from the First International Consensus Meeting. *Blood Rev.* 2020;41:100648.

screening cells. A follow-up antibody panel for any positive screening cell can confirm the presence of a pan-reactive antibody versus an alloantibody. In addition, reactivity at room temperature immediate spin hints at an IgM antibody, versus the 37°C-reactivity with antihuman globulin that is more typical of IgG. The use of an autocontrol then helps to distinguish an antibody to a high incidence antigen from an autoantibody. If the autocontrol is negative, it suggests the antibody in the plasma targets an antigen that is absent from the patient's red blood cells; thus, it is most likely an alloantibody being detected. Conversely, if the autocontrol is positive, it suggests there is an antibody in the plasma that reacts with the patient's own cells. In the presence of a positive autocontrol a reflex DAT is performed. With these basic tests, one can quickly identify a warm autoantibody, a cold autoantibody, and the need for further testing. As discussed previously, an autoantibody alone is not pathognomonic of an AIHA, as more typically they are found in nonhemolytic states. Clinical-pathologic correlation is essential.

The Direct Antiglobulin Test

The DAT helps distinguish immune from nonimmune hemolytic anemia. While the DAT should be performed to identify AIHA in patients with hemolytic anemia, it should not be used as a screening test for hemolytic anemia if the presence of hemolysis has not been established. The predictive value of a positive DAT is 83% in a patient with hemolytic anemia; however, this drops to 1.4% in a patient without hemolytic anemia.[4] In addition, positive DATs have been reported in 1% to 15% of hospitalized patients and fewer than 0.1% of healthy blood donors.[2]

Samples submitted for DAT testing should be collected in lavender topped EDTA tubes. The EDTA present in the tube chelates calcium in the sample and prevents in vitro fixation of complement.[5] The DAT is performed by first washing red blood cells to remove plasma containing free globulins (immunoglobulin and complement). Then antihuman globulin (AHG) reagent is added. In most laboratories, a polyspecific AHG is used initially, which detects both IgG and complement. The IgG is detected by an antibody targeting the IgG heavy chains (Fc portion), and complement is detected by an antibody to the C3d fragment of complement. If agglutination is observed following the addition of polyspecific AHG, then there is either IgG and/or complement present on the red cells. This agglutination can be assessed and scored by the strength of reactivity, which is usually proportional to the amount of bound protein.[5] If the results are positive with polyspecific AHG, tests with monospecific anti-IgG and anticomplement antisera are performed to appropriately distinguish the immune process involved.[5] Some laboratories do not use a polyspecific reagent and choose to test initially with monospecific anti-IgG and anticomplement antisera. Monospecific anticomplement often contains anti-C3b in addition to the anti-C3d used in polyspecific AHG. Although polyspecific AHG does not contain anti-IgM, complement deposition remains an indirect sign of prior IgM binding because IgM is a potent activator of complement.[6] It is important to remember that IgG1 and IgG3 are able to activate complement; however, most of the complement detected by the DAT is caused by IgM.[7] While some manufactures offer additional monospecific anticomplement antisera (anti-C3, -C3c, -C3d, -C4, -C4c), anti-C3d provides optimal detection of sensitization and is the only anticomplement antisera required by US FDA regulations.[8] With a positive result for the monospecific IgG reagent, an eluate is often performed. In the case of a WAIHA, the eluate will show pan-reactivity at 37°C with an AHG reagent, thus confirming that the patient's positive DAT is caused by an IgG antibody reacting against red cells at 37°C (see later in discussion for further discussion on eluates).

When no agglutination is observed, the DAT result is negative. A negative DAT result does not necessarily mean that the red cells have no attached globulin molecules. Known diagnostic pitfalls include IgG bound at a quantitative level below the threshold of sensitivity, low-affinity IgG, warm IgM, and IgA autoantibodies in addition to a myriad of technical issues. In manual tube testing, polyspecific and monospecific reagents detect 100 to 500 molecules of IgG per cell and 400 to 1100 molecules of complement per cell, but patients may still experience autoimmune hemolytic anemia when the coating molecules are below these levels of detection.[9] Testing with microcolumn and solid-phase methods is able to detect approximately 200 to 300 molecules of IgG per cell.[10] Novel tests, capable of detecting smaller amounts of antibodies, are discussed briefly later in discussion and in more detail in a subsequent article in this issue. Alternatively, the DAT result can be negative if low-affinity autoantibodies were present but then removed in the initial wash step. False-negative DAT results due to these low-affinity autoantibodies may be overcome by testing with low ionic strength saline (LISS) or performing the initial wash step using cold saline.[3] IgM autoantibodies that react with a thermal range close to 37°C (warm IgM) produce a rare but severe form of AIHA that also may be DAT-negative.[11] Testing with a dual DAT (DDAT), which is discussed in more detail later in discussion, aids in the identification of warm IgM autoantibodies that are typically missed by testing with a standard DAT only.[12] In addition, an IgA antibody will not be detected by a standard DAT; therefore, falsely negative-DATs occur in rare cases when the patient's hemolysis is due to IgA-mediated red blood cell destruction.[13,14] In 800 patients with DAT-negative hemolytic anemia, IgA alone was found on 2% of samples.[15]

As mentioned previously, a positive DAT result alone is not diagnostic of hemolytic anemia. The significance of a positive DAT result can only be interpreted in the context of a patient's medical history, including medication, pregnancy, transfusion, and hematopoietic transplantation history. It is also important to consider the specific testing method used when interpreting the results. In a comparative study of various DAT methods, Barcellini and colleagues found that the manual tube DAT method was the most specific but least sensitive test (0.87 and 0.43, respectively); whereas, other traditional DAT methods of microcolumn and solid phase showed reduced specificity but increased sensitivity (0.70 and 0.65, respectively).[16] Despite these limitations, additional serologic investigations, such as an eluate, can be helpful in the evaluation of an AIHA.

The Eluate

Elution frees antibody from sensitized red blood cells and recovers the antibody in a useable/testable/analyzable form, enabling the laboratory to determine the antibody's specificity. Like the antibody screen, this is accomplished by testing the freed antibodies present in the eluate against panel cells. An elution is typically only performed if the DAT is positive with monospecific anti-IgG antisera; however, one of the most common causes for AIHA associated with a negative DAT is RBC-bound IgG below the sensitivity threshold of the DAT, and it has been suggested that an eluate can be useful when there is a high clinical suspicion for AIHA and the DAT is negative.[15] In such a case, the eluate may be useful as it effectively concentrates the antibody present and therefore can gain sensitivity.

If the DAT was only positive for complement the eluate is likely to be nonreactive. If the DAT demonstrates the presence of IgG and the eluate reacts with all cells tested, including an autocontrol cell previously treated to remove bound antibody that on retesting demonstrates rebinding of the antibody, then an autoantibody is the most likely explanation. In this case, an adsorption should be performed to aid in identifying whether there are any alloantibodies present in addition to the pan-reactive autoanti-bodies (see later in discussion).

The eluate may also demonstrate the presence of alloantibodies that may have sensitized red blood cells in the context of a delayed hemolytic transfusion reaction or hemolytic disease of the fetus and newborn. Working closely with the transfusion medicine laboratory to determine transfusion history and with the obstetrics teams to determine pertinent pregnancy history often provides the clinical correlation neces-sary to appropriately interpret the significance of alloantibodies present in the eluate.

Adsorptions

It was mentioned above that pan-reactivity in the antibody screen and eluate is char-acteristic of warm AIHA. The presence of a pan-reactive autoantibody in the plasma increases the complexity of the transfusion laboratory's testing and results in signifi-cant time requirements to complete required pretransfusion testing, which must al-ways assess whether there are alloantibodies present in addition to any autoantibodies identified. The root of the problem is that the pan-reactive antibody can mask an underlying alloantibody. Additional testing using adsorptions is required to unmask such alloantibodies.

Adsorption is a method that removes autoantibody from the sample while preser-ving any alloantibodies that may exist. Fundamentally, a patient will only have an allo-antibody to an antigen that they lack; therefore, testing will use phenotypically similar red cells (ie, cells negative for the same antigens the patient lacks) to absorb autoan-tibody while leaving behind any alloantibody. Depending on the patient's medical his-tory, the absorbing cell can be an autologous red cell or an allogenic red cell. If there is no history that might result in an unclear red cell phenotype, such as recent transfu-sion, pregnancy, or stem cell transplantation, then autologous adsorption may be per-formed. If such a history does exist, allogenic red cell adsorption must be performed to prevent absorbing an alloantibody onto an unexpected antigen. Performing adsorp-tions to identify any underlying alloantibodies can increase testing time significantly, sometimes up to 8 to 12 hours.

Alternative to performing adsorption is to transfuse phenotypically matched blood. This approach is often utilized at institutions that do not have a reference laboratory in house; however, it is dependent on having an accurate phenotype. If the patient has not been transfused, serologic methods can identify the phenotype of the patient; however, in the context of recent transfusion, DNA-based methods are necessary to provide an accurate phenotype.

Warm Autoimmune Hemolytic Anemia

Most of the AIHA is caused by polyclonal warm reactive autoantibodies that react opti-mally at 37°C. In making the diagnosis of WAIHA, a clinically significant cold reactive antibody should be excluded. WAIHA is classically defined by reactivity at 37° C and a DAT that is positive for IgG with or without complement. However, a high thermal amplitude IgM or IgA can also result in WAIHA.[3,11,15] In IgG-positive WAIHA, the elution is typically pan-reactive with all cells tested, including the autocontrol.

In approximately one-third of patients with WAIHA, agglutination is also detected at room temperature due to nonpathologic IgM antibodies; however, these cold-reacting agglutinins (CA) have titers less than 64 at 4°C and are nonreactive at warmer temper-atures of 30 to 37°C. Because the CA titer is <64, they are not considered clinically significant and the patient does not meet defined criteria for CAS or CAD in addition to WAIHA.[2,6] This is important to distinguish from the more severe and rare form of mixed-type AIHA given the difference in prognosis and treatment approach.

IgM-mediated WAIHA is associated with IgM autoantibodies that react at 37°C and may portend a poorer prognosis with rapid progression of fatal hemolysis noted.[2,11] These autoantibodies tend to cause spontaneous agglutination in the DAT, making identification a challenge. Traditional testing methods can overcome the interference caused by a warm IgM by treatment with dithiothreitol (DTT) or 2-mercaptoethanol (2-ME), which disrupts the disulfide bonds of IgM molecules and enables controls to be appropriately evaluated. It is important to distinguish warm IgM from clinically significant cold agglutinins, which can be easily done by titration studies. Warm IgM often has low titers of less than 64 at 4°C, which makes the distinction from typical CAS and CAD.[5] Of note some authors would still consider this to be "low titer high thermal amplitude" and a part of the spectrum of CAS/CAD. Below in the novel testing section, we discuss the dual DAT, which is another method to identify warm IgM.

Cold Agglutinin Syndrome and Cold Agglutinin Disease

Clinically significant cold agglutinins are usually IgM-mediated with complement as the only protein detected on the DAT. As in vitro testing demonstrates that IgM binding is optimal at colder temperatures, it is assumed that in vivo IgM binding occurs in the peripheral circulation and causes complement activation. As the cells are circulated to warmer central regions of the vasculature, the IgM dissociates, and the bound complement remains.

CAS and CAD both have a DAT positive for complement (and negative for IgG) with a cold agglutinin titer greater than 64 when tested at 4°C. Of note, while the accepted threshold for diagnosis is 64, many experts consider a range between 64 and 512 to be equivocal and a titer more than 512 to be clinically significant.[17] The titer is determined by testing serial dilutions of patient serum and each dilution's ability to agglutinate red blood cells. The titer is the inverse of the highest dilution at which agglutination occurs. As such, the titer reflects the concentration and avidity of the antibody. Usually, the titer needs to be ordered separately and results are reported separately from the DAT. Depending on how the test has been validated, some institutions may report the IgM titer based on critical thresholds, such as less than 64, 64 to 512, or greater than 512. Therefore, a low titer would be reported as less than 64.

Patients with CAS have a known associated condition, for example, autoimmune disorders, infection, clinical or radiologic evidence of B-cell lymphoma, or another malignancy. On the other hand, patients with CAD lack an associated condition; however, they may have a B-cell clonal lymphoproliferative disorder detectable in blood or marrow, but no clinical or radiological evidence of malignancy.[6]

Cold agglutinins that are clinically significant for causing hemolysis are usually present at high titers (greater than 512) when tested at 4°C and they often react at 30°C; however, it has been noted that some clinically significant cold agglutinins may have a lower titer. Thermal amplitude testing identifies the highest temperature at which the antibody will bind to an antigen and whether the cold IgM autoantibody will be clinically significant at relevant temperatures. The thermal amplitude test is performed at 4°C, 22°C, 30°C, and 37°C to determine the temperatures at which the cold autoantibody is reactive. Cold antibodies that are reactive at temperatures less than 30°C are not considered to be clinically significant in most situations. When the IgM antibody reactions at greater than 30°C, it may be causing hemolysis; therefore, it has the potential to be clinically significant even at a low titer. As such, thermal amplitude testing is best used when a hemolytic patient has a DAT positive for complement only and cold agglutinins are present at low titers because thermal amplitude testing identifies the "low titer high thermal amplitude" cold agglutinins that might be missed when using greater than 64 or greater than 512 as a cut off for clinically significant cold agglutinins. It is important to remember that to determine the true thermal amplitude or titer of a suspected cold agglutinin, the specimen must be collected and maintained at 37°C until the serum and red cells are separated to avoid in vitro autoadsorption of the IgM autoantibody.[5]

Mixed-Type Autoimmune Hemolytic Anemia

While there is a set of patients that have both WAIHA and nonpathogenic cold antibodies (discussed in the WAIHA section above), there is a smaller group of patients that have both WAIHA and a pathogenic cold component. This latter group is often referred to as "mixed-type" AIHA. Typically, mixed-type AIHA will have a DAT positive for both IgG and complement. In addition, there is evidence of both a warm IgG antibody and a cold antibody with a thermal amplitude $\geq$30°C.[6]

Usually both IgG and complement are detected in the DAT of mixed forms, but it's been reported that IgG, complement, or IgA alone were detected in mixed-type AIHA.[2] As with other IgG-mediated AIHAs, the eluate is usually pan-reactive. Unique to this group of patients, however, is that the adsorption testing necessary to detect the presence of underlying alloantibodies must be performed at both 4°C and 37°C.[5]

Paroxysmal Cold Hemoglobinuria

PCH is the rarest form of DAT-positive AIHA. It often presents secondary to a viral infection in young children. As such, the classic biphasic (also termed bithermic) hemolysin may only be transiently detectable. This hemolysin associated with PCH is a cold-reactive IgG antibody capable of binding complement. As with CAS/CAD, the antibody binds in the colder periphery, and complement is fixed before movement to warmer body parts. Activation of the classical complement pathway occurs after warming to 37°C in the central circulation at which time the IgG dissociates.[18] Therefore, routine DAT results will often only be positive for the complement. These patients typically do not have IgG positivity on their red blood cell surface and no evidence of autoantibody activity in the serum or the eluate made from the DAT-positive cells.

Testing for PCH with a Donath–Landsteiner (DL) test is suggested for patients with a positive DAT result due to complement alone with demonstrable hemoglobinemia or hemoglobinuria. A DL tests the patient's serum at different temperatures to mimic the presumed in vivo activation of the biphasic antibody: constantly cold, a bithermic stage that begins cold and finishes warm, and constantly warm. In each temperature set, there are 3 tubes: a tube with patient plasma only, a tube with patient plasma and additional donor plasma, and a negative control without patient plasma. The donor plasma supplements complement levels that may be low due to consumption in a patient with active hemolysis. If the DL test demonstrates hemolysis in the biphasic set of tests alone, it is diagnostic of PCH, as seen in **Fig. 1**. This is a cumbersome test with a stringent requirement for the patient sample to remain at 37° C; therefore, it is typically only performed at in-house reference laboratories.

Additional Testing

Autoantibodies most often have broad specificities leading to the classic pan-reactive testing described above; whereas, in other cases, specificity to single antigen types can be seen. Regardless of the specificities of the antibodies, distinguishing an alloantibody versus an autoantibody remains essential. This is typically done by using commercial antigen typing reagents (polyclonal and monoclonal antibodies) to determine if the patient possesses the antigen to which the antibody is specific. This is analyzed in combination with the autocontrol as in some cases patients express only partial antigen molecules and can make true alloantibodies against the nonexpressed portions. Additional genetic testing using single nucleotide polymorphism

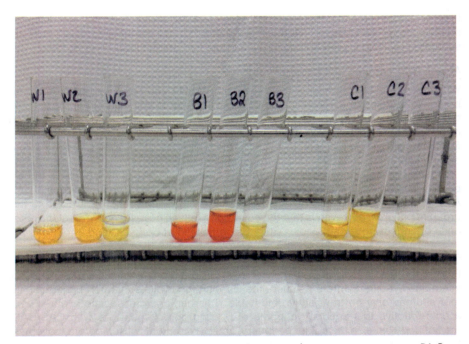

Fig. 1. Positive Donath–Landsteiner Test. W1–W3 are tested at warm temperatures; B1–3 are the biphasic tubes, and C1–3 are the cold tubes. For each set, tube 1 contains patient plasma, tube 2 contains patient plasma and additional donor plasma in case the patient's complement levels are low, and tube 3 is a negative control without patient plasma. A positive test demonstrates hemolysis that occurs only in the biphasic tubes (B1 and B2) and negative in the negative control (B3). (*Courtesy of* Mayo Clinic Laboratories, Mayo Clinic, Rochester, MN.)

(SNP) analysis with commercial arrays or gene sequencing at reference laboratories can also be helpful to confirm such findings.

Monocyte Monolayer Assay

Occasionally, an allo- or autoantibody is present that is of unclear clinical significance. The MMA is designed to assess the clinical relevance of antibodies. This is done by mixing the patient's plasma with red blood cells expressing the antigen to which the antibodies have specificity. Third party donor monocytes are added and both opsonization and phagocytosis of red blood cells are assessed microscopically. If more than 5% of the red blood cells are either tethered to a monocyte or phagocytosed, then the antibody is considered clinically significant. Although not always done, it is possible to use the patient's own cells rather than donor red blood cells.

Drug-Induced Hemolytic Anemia

Drug-induced hemolytic anemia (DIHA) is covered elsewhere in this issue and will not be discussed at length. It is important to be aware, however, that the findings can mimic a standard warm autoantibody typical of AIHA or show no reactivity. This is due to the neo-epitopes target and the immune mechanisms that generate the antibodies in this underrecognized entity. It is necessary to obtain a detailed clinical history with a clear timeline in relation to the start of hemolysis and the start and stop time of new drugs in the weeks and months preceding hemolysis. Specialized testing methodologies can help confirm suspicions of DIHA.

Novel Direct Antiglobulin Test Testing

Additional variations of DAT are discussed elsewhere in this addition of the journal but are briefly mentioned here. Novel tests, typically only performed in reference laboratories, are capable of detecting smaller amounts of antibodies bound to the patient's red blood cells compared with the standard manual tube DAT testing; however, positivity in these novel tests must be interpreted with caution given their higher sensitivities and lower specificities.

Flow cytometry provides a simple and low-cost method to detect immunoglobulin and complement bound to red blood cells; however, positive results have limited stand-alone value. While a standard tube DAT identifies IgG on red blood cells in 1 in 1400 healthy donors, flow cytometry is so sensitive that it can be positive for IgG-bound red blood cells in most, if not all, individuals.[2,19,20] Recall that a manual tube DAT will result as positive if a minimum of 100 to 500 molecules of IgG are present per red blood cell. Flow cytometry is so sensitive that it will detect as few as 30 to 40 molecules of IgG per red blood cell.[20] Therefore, the use of flow cytometry may be useful in the DAT-negative AIHA patient in which there is an extremely high level of clinical suspicion. Specifically, the flow DAT can aid in the detection of IgM AIHA and can subclass IgG molecules to assess the risk of complement-mediated intravascular hemolysis.[21] The extreme sensitivity of the test necessitates careful clinical correlation with any positive results.

Mitogen stimulated DAT (MS-DAT) is a functional and quantitative method that detects red blood cell antibodies that may be too few for standard DAT methods to detect. A culture of a patient's whole blood is performed in the presence of IL-6 and mitogens, which results in an amplification of antibody production and significantly increases the IgG bound to autologous red blood cells compared with unstimulated cultures.[22] Compared with standard manual tube DAT and microcolumn/solid-phase DATs, the MS-DAT is the least specific but the most sensitive test (0.59 and 0.88, respectively).[16] Although highly sensitive, the utility of MS-DAT is limited to patients not on steroid therapy, as steroids affect the in vitro lymphocyte capability to respond to mitogen stimulation and may result in false-negative results.[23]

There are numerous other novel methods to identify the presence of antiglobulin and/or complement on red blood cells. These include the immunoradiometric assay (IRMA), the complement fixation antibody consumption test, the enzyme-linked immunoassay test (ELAT), as well as the enzyme-linked immunosorbent assay (ELISA).[24–27] While these tests each may identify red blood cell-bound antibody, the quantity of bound antibody remains only one of the many factors influencing the degree of erythrocyte destruction, and as such, the manual tube DAT remains the gold standard to be interpreted in the patient with hemolysis.[19,20] However, as echoed by Barcellini, Petz, and Garratty, no single test is optimal in the diagnosis of AIHA.

The dual DAT (DDAT) method was developed because warm IgM AIHA is a serious disease, yet laboratory testing was inadequate at identifying IgM autoantibodies. The presence of IgM is often implicated when complement is detected in the DAT result; however, direct identification of IgM in the DAT has been limited by multiple factors. The use of anti-human IgM is limited due to spontaneous red blood cell agglutination, which results in invalid test controls, and as such, there remains a lack of standardized anti-IgM reagents. The DDAT bypasses this limitation by performing 2 stages of sensitization with IgG rabbit anti-human IgM and then IgG goat anti-rabbit IgG. First, the DAT cells are incubated with a rabbit IgG antibody that is specific to human IgM. The cells are washed, and any unbound antibody is removed. A second incubation step occurs following the addition of a goat IgG with anti-rabbit IgG specificity. The presence of agglutination following the dual incubations indicates that the original DAT cells had human IgM bound to them.[12] By controlling the temperatures of the incubation and wash steps, the dual DAT method enables one to identify IgM bound in vivo to the red blood cells without invalidating testing.

SUMMARY

AIHA is a series of clinical entities diagnosed by standard and specialized transfusion laboratory testing used in the appropriate clinical setting. In patients with confirmed hemolysis, an ABO type and screen with a DAT can often diagnose the standard WAIHA. Additional specialized testing such as cold agglutinin titers and the Donath–Landsteiner test for biphasic hemagglutinins can further define the presence of more rare entities such as CAS/CAD or PCH. Other specialized testing such as enhanced DATs and testing for drug-induced hemolytic anemias can also be useful in the appropriate setting. An open dialogue and consultation between the clinician and laboratorian can often lend efficiency and specificity to the workup while correlating the clinical history with the laboratory findings.

CLINICS CARE POINTS

- Standard tests such as ABO typing and antibody screening along with a DAT are the intial starting point for testing for AIHA.
- Specialized testing such as sensitive DAT testing should only be performed with a known history of AIHA.
- All testing should be interpreted within the clinical context.

DISCLOSURE

The authors have nothing to disclose.

REFERENCES

1. Barcellini W, Fattizzo B, Zaninoni A, et al. Clinical heterogeneity and predictors of outcome in primary autoimmune hemolytic anemia: a GIMEMA study of 308 patients. Blood 2014;124(19):2930–6.
2. Petz LD, Garratty G. Immune hemolytic anemias. 2nd Ed ed. Philadelphia: Churchill-Livingstone; 2004.
3. Barcellini W. Pitfalls in the diagnosis of autoimmune haemolytic anaemia. Blood Transfus 2015;13(1):3–5.
4. Kaplan HS, Garratty G. Predictive value of direct antiglobulin test results. Diagn Med 1985;8:29–32.
5. Borge PD, Mansfield PM. The Positive Direct Antiglobulin Test and Immune-Mediated Hemolysis. In: Cohn CS, Delaney M, Johnson ST, et al, editors. Technical manual. 20th ed. Bethesda, MD: AABB; 2020. p. 429–78.
6. Jager U, Barcellini W, Broome CM, et al. Diagnosis and treatment of autoimmune hemolytic anemia in adults: Recommendations from the First International Consensus Meeting. Blood Rev 2020;41:100648.
7. Meulenbroek EM, de Haas M, Brouwer C, et al. Complement deposition in autoimmune hemolytic anemia is a footprint for difficult-to-detect IgM autoantibodies. Haematologica 2015;100(11):1407–14.

8. Garratty G, Petz LD. The significance of red cell bound complement components in development of standards and quality assurance for the anti-complement components of antiglobulin sera. Transfusion 1976;16(4):297–306.

9. Coombs RR, Mourant AE, Race RR. A new test for the detection of weak and incomplete Rh agglutinins. Br J Exp Pathol 1945;26:255–66.

10. Dubarry M, Charron C, Habibi B, et al. Quantitation of immunoglobulin classes and subclasses of autoantibodies bound to red cells in patients with and without hemolysis. Transfusion 1993;33(6):466–71.

11. Arndt PA, Leger RM, Garratty G. Serologic findings in autoimmune hemolytic anemia associated with immunoglobulin M warm autoantibodies. Transfusion 2009; 49(2):235–42.

12. Bartolmas T, Salama A. A dual antiglobulin test for the detection of weak or non-agglutinating immunoglobulin M warm autoantibodies. Transfusion 2010;50(5): 1131–4.

13. Villa MA, Fantini NN, Revelli N, et al. IgA autoimmune haemolytic anaemia in a pregnant woman. Blood Transfus 2014;12(3):443–5.

14. Bajpayee A, Dubey A, Verma A, et al. A report of a rare case of autoimmune haemolytic anaemia in a patient with Hodgkin's disease in whom routine serology was negative. Blood Transfus 2014;12(Suppl 1):s299–301.

15. Leger RM, Co A, Hunt P, et al. Attempts to support an immune etiology in 800 patients with direct antiglobulin test-negative hemolytic anemia. Immunohematology 2010;26(4):156–60.

16. Barcellini W, Revelli N, Imperiali FG, et al. Comparison of traditional methods and mitogen-stimulated direct antiglobulin test for detection of anti-red blood cell autoimmunity. Int J Hematol 2010;91(5):762–9.

17. Swiecicki PL, Hegerova LT, Gertz MA. Cold agglutinin disease. Blood 2013; 122(7):1114–21.

18. Berentsen S, Barcellini W. Autoimmune Hemolytic Anemias. N Engl J Med 2021; 385(15):1407–19.

19. Garratty G. Effect of cell-bound proteins on the in vivo survival of circulating blood cells. Gerontology 1991;37(1–3):68–94.

20. Garratty G. The significance of IgG on the red cell surface. Transfus Med Rev 1987;1(1):47–57.

21. Garratty G, Arndt PA. Applications of flow cytofluorometry to red blood cell immunology. Cytometry 1999;38(6):259–67.

22. Barcellini W, Clerici G, Montesano R, et al. In vitro quantification of anti-red blood cell antibody production in idiopathic autoimmune haemolytic anaemia: effect of mitogen and cytokine stimulation. Br J Haematol 2000;111(2):452–60.

23. Briggs WA, Eustace J, Gimenez LF, et al. Lymphocyte suppression by glucocorticoids with cyclosporine, tacrolimus, pentoxifylline, and mycophenolic acid. J Clin Pharmacol 1999;39(2):125–30.

24. Bodensteiner D, Brown P, Skikne B, et al. The enzyme-linked immunosorbent assay: accurate detection of red blood cell antibodies in autoimmune hemolytic anemia. Am J Clin Pathol 1983;79(2):182–5.

25. Greenwalt TJ, Domino MM, Dumaswala UJ. An enzyme-linked antiglobulin test to quantify nanogram quantities of IgG on polystyrene microspheres. Vox Sang 1992;63(4):272–5.

26. Gilliland BC, Leddy JP, Vaughan JH. The detection of cell-bound antibody on complement-coated human red cells. J Clin Invest 1970;49(5):898–906.

27. Jeje MO, Blajchman MA, Steeves K, et al. Quantitation of red cell-associated IgG using an immunoradiometric assay. Transfusion 1984;24(6):473–6.

DAT-Negative Autoimmune Hemolytic Anemia

Karen Rodberg, MBA, MT(ASCP)SBB

KEYWORDS

- AIHA • DAT • DAT-Negative • Coombs-negative • Autoimmune hemolytic anemia
- Low-affinity antibody • Super Coombs

KEY POINTS

- IgG on red blood cells (RBCs) of patients with AIHA may be difficult to detect if the quantity is low or if the IgG is of low affinity.
- AIHA can be caused by IgA or IgM autoantibodies not detected by routine serologic reagents.
- More sensitive methods may be needed to detect immunoglobulins coating a patient's red blood cells.
- These more sensitive methods are only available at a few immunohematology reference laboratories.

INTRODUCTION

Laboratory testing is often used to support clinical diagnoses. For patients with signs and symptoms of autoimmune hemolytic anemia (AIHA), the laboratory test most often used to confirm this diagnosis is the direct Coombs test, more accurately called the direct antiglobulin test (DAT). In a clinical laboratory, this test is performed by the Blood Bank Department and is usually conducted using a polyspecific antihuman globulin reagent. If positive, reflex testing is performed using anti-IgG and anti-complement reagents. If one, or both, of these tests, is positive, it tends to support the diagnosis of AIHA.

On occasion, the DAT is negative while the clinical picture clearly suggests an extrinsic mechanism of red blood cell (RBC) destruction, that is, transfused RBCs and autologous RBCs are being cleared at approximately the same rate. Patients with DAT Negative AIHA will also respond to typical therapeutic measures such as steroids or splenectomy. Additional testing for DAT negative AIHA may be performed by specialized laboratories to investigate if there is low-affinity IgG or low quantity of IgG coating a patient's RBCs, or whether there is complement, IgM or IgA coating the

Immunohematology Reference Labs, Northern and Southern California, American Red Cross, 100 Red Cross Circle, Pomona, CA 91768, USA
E-mail address: Karen.Rodberg@redcross.org

Hematol Oncol Clin N Am 36 (2022) 307–313
https://doi.org/10.1016/j.hoc.2021.11.004
0889-8588/22/© 2021 Elsevier Inc. All rights reserved.

hemonc.theclinics.com

patient's red blood cells.[1] If any of these tests is positive, it tends to support the diagnosis of AIHA. Our laboratory is one of the few in the United States that can perform this specialized testing. Hematologists often order this panel of testing as "super Coombs."

BACKGROUND

Dr George Garratty was a world-renowned immunohematologist, author, teacher, and lecturer about autoimmune hemolytic anemia. Dr Garratty started his career in London, England, working for Sir John Dacie and Dr Patrick Mollison, 2 world leaders in the field of immunohematology. After immigrating to the United States, he did research at the University of California, San Francisco for a decade. In 1978 he became the Scientific Director of the American Red Cross, and relocated to Southern California. He held that position until his death in 2014. Along with Dr Lawrence Petz, he authored a textbook[2] on the subject of immune hemolytic anemia in 1980 and published a revised edition in 2004. Over the course of many years, as Scientific Director at the American Red Cross, samples were submitted to Dr Garratty's laboratory for evaluation to see if immunoglobulin could be detected to explain the patient's hemolytic anemia. After testing hundreds of samples, a particular panel of tests became standardized in our laboratory as determined by those found to be most useful in this patient population.

QUANTITY OF ANTIBODY ON RED BLOOD CELLS

In the early seventies, Gilliland and coworkers[3] first suggested that the amount of antibody on RBCs of patients with AIHA might be too low to be detected by the routine DAT. Normal individuals typically have less than 25 to 120 molecules of IgG/RBC (as determined by a complement-fixation antibody consumption test, which can detect antigen–antibody reactions that cannot be visualized by agglutination or hemolysis) but some subjects studied had much higher levels, yet, had a negative DAT using anti-IgG.[4] One possible explanation they advanced was that the IgG was not distributed equally on all RBCs in circulation. RBCs accumulate IgG as the cells age, so older RBCs tend to have more IgG/RBC than younger RBCs. Kay[5] proposed that in normal individuals, RBCs are removed from circulation due to an autoantibody to senescent cell antigen (SCA). At a certain point (eg, 120 days for normal individuals) these RBCs are then removed by macrophages. As only a small percentage of circulating RBCs (the senescent cells) would have a large quantity of IgG on them, the DAT may not be positive because the RBCs are not close enough together to cause cross-linking.

Another explanation is that the nature of the IgG on the RBCs differed among individuals. Our laboratory sees positive DATs in approximately 1 of 1400 healthy blood donors[6] with no apparent pathology. Masouredis and coworkers[6] studied a similar population of healthy donors and eluted 2 kinds of IgG from their RBCs, one being autoantibody to red cell antigens and the other being auto-anti-idiotype which targeted the IgG autoantibody. They proposed that this second autoantibody protected the donor's RBCs from destruction. So, although the amount of IgG on their RBCs was large, there was no abnormal degree of hemolysis.

LOW-AFFINITY IgG

When a routine DAT is performed, the patient's RBCs are washed with large volumes of saline to remove all residual plasma that could neutralize the anti-IgG reagent used to perform the DAT. Typically, this saline is at room temperature (RT) but occasionally it is at 37°C (eg, if a cold agglutinin is present and warm washes are used to remove the cold agglutinin). In one study of 22 patients by Garratty and associates[7] low-affinity IgG was able to be detected if the RBCs were washed with cold (4°C) saline or low ionic strength saline (LISS) instead of RT or 37°C saline. This same phenomenon can occur in some samples if the washed RBCs are allowed to stand at RT before anti-IgG is added, which can happen in a laboratory setting whereby interruptions are constant.

OTHER IMMUNOGLOBULINS

Other less frequent immunoglobulins such as anti-IgA and anti-IgM can be found coating RBCs in some patients with DAT-negative AIHA. Commercial polyspecific anti-globulin sera will detect IgG and C3 on RBCs. Anti-IgA and anti-IgM standardized for use with RBCs are not commercially available but can be prepared from other sources.

IgA AIHA has a clinical picture similar to IgG warm AIHA, but the DAT is often nega-tive when performed with standard antiglobulin sera. Patients typically respond to the same therapies as those with IgG warm AIHA. There have been numerous reports of patients with IgA AIHA (eg, Sokol, and colleagues[8]), but these are still rare occurrences.

IgM warm AIHA is even more rare, but can be severe, even fatal due to significant complement activation and C5 convertase formation. While most IgM AIHA is due to pathologic cold autoantibody of broad thermal range that is reacting at 30 to 37°C, warm IgM AIHA is difficult to diagnose because the serology is often unremark-able, in that only very weak reactivity may be noted in antibody detection tests. Both pathologic IgM cold autoantibodies and warm IgM autoantibodies present with com-plement coating the patient's RBCs. For this reason, some patients with warm IgM AIHA are misdiagnosed as having cold agglutinin disease (CAD) or paroxysmal cold hemoglobinuria (PCH).

Arndt and colleagues[9] reported on 49 cases of IgM warm AIHA tested over a period of 25 years. In this series 44 patients had C3 on their RBCs, 23 of whom had C3 only, and 14 had detectable IgM on their RBCs, 3 of whom had IgM alone. The RBCs in the ma-jority (78%) of these patients with IgM warm AIHA exhibited spontaneous agglutination; that is, their well-washed RBCs agglutinated in an inert diluent such as saline or 6% al-bumin. Spontaneous agglutination differs from cold agglutination in that it is not reversed by washing the RBCs with warm saline or incubating the sample at 37°C before washing the RBCs. Spontaneously agglutinated RBCs can be treated with 0.01 M dithiothreitol (DTT) to disrupt the IgM pentamers before testing, but if DTT-treated RBCs are used in the assay with anti-IgM they often give false-negative results. In this series, 94% of the patients' sera directly agglutinated test RBCs at 37°C. Titra-tions performed at 37°C, 30°C, 22°C, and 4°C may be used to determine the optimal temperature of the agglutinin to distinguish between cold and warm IgM autoantibodies.

COMPLEMENT

Complement-coated RBCs can be detected by a routine DAT performed with poly-specific antiglobulin serum or anti-C3 reagents. It is important for diagnosing AIHA to use an anti-C3 rich in anti-C3d. While it is not uncommon to find complement in small quantities on the RBCs of patients and normal individuals, strongly coated RBCs are usually associated with pathology. But similar to the situation whereby IgG is difficult to detect, complement can be hard to detect in some patients with AIHA if the anti-complement reagent lacks the ideal quantity of anti-C3d.

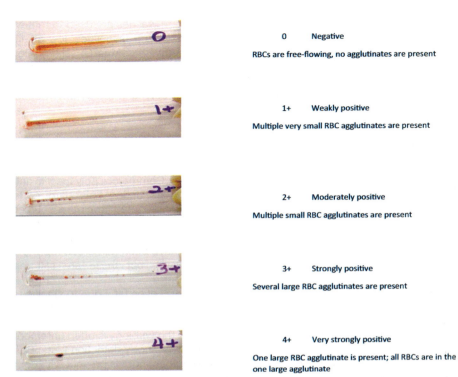

0   Negative

RBCs are free-flowing, no agglutinates are present

1+   Weakly positive

Multiple very small RBC agglutinates are present

2+   Moderately positive

Multiple small RBC agglutinates are present

3+   Strongly positive

Several large RBC agglutinates are present

4+   Very strongly positive

One large RBC agglutinate is present; all RBCs are in the one large agglutinate

Fig. 1. Grading of RBC agglutination reactions, from negative (0) no agglutination to strong (4+) agglutination: 0 Negative: RBCs are free-flowing, no agglutinates are present. 1+ Weakly positive: Multiple very small RBC agglutinates are present. 2+ Moderately positive: Multiple small RBC agglutinates are present. 3+ Strongly positive: Several large RBC agglutinates are present. 4+ Very strongly positive: One large RBC agglutinate is present; all RBCs are in the one large agglutinate.

METHODS USED
Detection of IgG

Commercial anti-IgG is used by several techniques in our assay. We test by conventional tube method with 2 sources of anti-IgG (rabbit and monoclonal). We use these same anti-IgG sera with the cold LISS wash technique. We use the rabbit source of anti-IgG in the direct and indirect Polybrene tests.

- Conventional DAT with anti-IgG: RBCs are washed manually with 4 washes of RT phosphate-buffered saline (PBS) and prepared as a 3% to 5% RBC suspension, similar to that used in routine Blood Banking techniques. One drop of RBCs is added to the tube and 2 drops of the anti-IgG reagent are added and immediately centrifuged for the calibrated time for that serologic centrifuge. The tubes are then read for agglutination macroscopically and microscopically (if negative macro) and results graded for the strength of reactivity (negative to 4+) and recorded (**Fig. 1**)
- Another RBC suspension is prepared using cold (4°C) LISS prepared according to Low and Messeter,[10] but ice-cold saline can be used alternatively. The RBC washes are performed in a refrigerated centrifuge to keep them at 4°C

throughout testing. One drop of 3% to 5% cold RBCs and 2 drops of cold anti-IgG are mixed and centrifuged. The tubes are read for agglutination macroscopically and if negative then microscopically and results graded for the strength of reactivity and recorded. An inert control, for example, 6% albumin, must be tested in parallel to assure that a positive result is not due to a cold agglutinin. If the negative control is reactive, the test is invalid.

- If no IgG is detected by either method above, we perform direct and indirect Polybrene testing according to the Lalezari[11] method. Polybrene is a polymer that brings RBCs very close together so that cross-linking can occur if antibody present on the RBCs can react with several RBCs in proximity. Results are read for direct agglutination and then taken through the indirect antiglobulin phase using anti-IgG. Results are graded and recorded.

Detection of Complement

A non-commercial source of anti-C3, rich in anti-C3d, is used for our assay. This in-house source of anti-C3 was prepared by injecting rabbits with purified proteins and then standardized for use in serology by testing various dilutions made with 6% bovine serum albumin. The optimal dilution was selected for the assay.

- RBCs previously prepared to a 3% to 5% suspension by washing at RT with saline are used. One drop of RBCs and 2 drops of anti-C3 are mixed and immediately centrifuged for the calibrated time. The tubes are read for agglutination macroscopically and microscopically (if neg macro) and results graded for the strength of reactivity and recorded. Negatives may be incubated for an additional 5 minutes and recentrifuged.

Detection of IgA or IgM

Anti-IgA and anti-IgM reagents have been standardized for use in serologic tests by preparing IgA and IgM-coated RBCs using chromic chloride. Optimal dilutions of anti-IgA and anti-IgM are then used in the assay.

- RBCs previously prepared to a 3% to 5% suspension by washing at RT with saline are used. One drop of RBCs and 2 drops of anti-IgA or anti-IgM are mixed and immediately centrifuged for the calibrated time. The tubes are read for agglutination macroscopically and microscopically (if neg macro) and results graded for the strength of reactivity and recorded. Tests may be incubated at RT for an additional 5 minutes and centrifuged again if so standardized for that lot of anti-IgA or anti-IgM.

OTHER TEST METHODS EVALUATED BUT NOT CURRENTLY USED IN OUR LABORATORY

Historically other methods including flow cytometry, concentrated eluates, monocyte monolayer assay, direct PEG, column agglutination test for DAT, and direct enzyme-linked antiglobulin test have been used. However, the value of these assays did not show enough efficacy to be included in routine testing or were too technically demanding to be practical.

DISCUSSION

Dr Garratty's laboratory gathered data over a 7-year period[12] on 398 samples sent for investigation of DAT-negative AIHA. These data were used to determine the percentage of patients whose RBCs reacted by at least one method. In this series, 48% of the samples studied were positive by at least one method. IgG was detected in 55 cases (14%) by standard technique but in 64 cases (16%) using cold LISS wash, C3 was detected in 148 cases (37%), IgA was detected in 9 cases (2%), but IgM was not detected in any of these cases. Direct Polybrene also detected IgG in 28 cases (8%). Although 48% of the samples gave a positive test result, 52% did not. The study concluded that some of the differences in the reference laboratory versus the referring laboratory may have been due to technique; however, there were many positive DATs due to differences in the reagents used in the DAT-negative hemolytic anemia panel of tests which are unavailable in a hospital Blood Bank laboratory.

The study was expanded in 2010 to include 800 patients in a 12-year span.[13] The techniques used in analyzing these specimens were the same as those described earlier in this paper in 635 (79%) of the specimens; however, the cold LISS wash test and the Polybrene tests were not performed on some samples if the antiglobulin sera or the anti-C3 gave a positive result. Positive DAT results were obtained in 431 (54%) specimens by at least one method. In fact, 48% of the samples had detectable IgG or C3, or both. This study concluded that no one method was optimal.

Our immunohematology reference laboratory has been testing samples submitted for DAT-negative hemolytic anemia investigation for more than 15 years in accordance with our protocols under Dr Garratty. Once the panel of tests was determined and reagents standardized, the performance of the test could be performed by any trained clinical laboratory scientist. Our degree of positivity of results is similar to the extensive study we performed in 2010. We continue with the panel of tests determined to be most helpful and relatively easy to perform. The battery of tests described seems to be the most efficient approach in investigating a situation of a DAT-negative AIHA. Often the reactivity observed is a weak positive result with one or more reagents, which has been useful to Hematologists submitting samples to our laboratory.

An important aspect to consider when sending samples to our laboratory is the confounding effect of recent transfusion. . The presence of transfused RBCs compromises the test results because nonautologous RBCs from normal donors are present. As the stated purpose of the test is to confirm a patient's diagnosis of AIHA, the ideal sample for this test is whole blood from a patient who has not been recently transfused. As such, early suspicion that a patient may have DAT-AIHA should prompt the clinician to send a sample for analysis to our laboratory before transfusing the patient.

SUMMARY

DAT-AIHA can pose a diagnostic challenge. Our laboratory has developed extensive and validated testing to support the clinician's suspicion, and potentially affect therapeutic decisions. In the last 15 years, we have analyzed well over 1000 samples. We continue to collaborate with regional and national medical centers in service to these challenging patients. Samples for investigation may be submitted to our laboratory through your practicing hospital's Blood Bank Department.

CLINICS CARE POINTS

- A positive result with any of the antiglobulin reagents can help support a diagnosis of autoimmune hemolytic anemia. But, even with sensitive test methods, our experience shows negative DAT results in approximately 50% of the samples tested.

DISCLOSURE

The author has nothing to disclose.

REFERENCES

1. Garratty G. Immune hemolytic anemia associated with negative routine serology. Semin Hematol 2005;42:156–64.
2. Petz LD, Garratty G. Immune hemolytic anemias. 2nd edition. Elsevier; 2004.
3. Gilliland BC, Baxter E, Evans RS. Red cell antibodies in acquired hemolytic anemia with negative antiglobulin serum tests. N Engl J Med 1971;285:252–6.
4. Garratty G. The significance of IgG on the red cell surface. Trans Med Rev 1987; 1:47–57.
5. Kay MMB. Senescent cell antigen: a red cell aging antigen. In: Garratty G, editor. Red cell antigens and antibodies. American Association of Blood Banks; 1986. p. 35.
6. Masouredis SP, Branks MJ, Victoria EJ. Antiidiotypic IgG crossreactive with Rh alloantibodies in red cell autoimmunity. Blood 1987;70:710–5.
7. Garratty G, Arndt P, Nance S. Low affinity autoantibodies – a cause of false negative direct antiglobulin tests (abstract). Book of Abstracts of the ISBT/AABB Joint Congress; 1990. p. 87.
8. Sokol RJ, Booker DJ, Stamps R, et al. IgA red cell autoantibodies and autoimmune hemolysis. Transfusion 1997;37:175–81.
9. Arndt P, Leger R, Garratty G. Serologic findings in autoimmune hemolytic anemia associated with immunoglobulin M warm autoantibodies. Immunohematology 2009;49:235–42.
10. Low B, Messeter L. Antiglobulin test in low-ionic strength salt solution for rapid antibody screening and cross-matching. Vox Sang 1974;26:53–61.
11. Lalezari P, Jiang AF. The manual polybrene test: A simple and rapid procedure for detection of red cell antibodies. Transfusion 1980;20:206–11.
12. Garratty G, Leger RM, Hunt P, et al. Serological investigation of a large series of direct antiglobulin test-negative hemolytic anemias; SP313. AABB Suppl 2004; 44:121A–2A.
13. Leger RM, Co A, Hunt P, et al. Attempts to support an immune etiology in 800 patients with direct antiglobulin test-negative hemolytic anemia. Immunohematology 2010;26:156–60.

Autoimmune Hemolytic Anemia: Diagnosis and Differential Diagnosis

Caleb J. Scheckel, DO*, Ronald S. Go, MD

KEYWORDS

- Anemia • Autoimmune • Cold agglutinin disease • Coombs test • Hemolysis
- Hereditary • Warm AIHA

KEY POINTS

- While the differential diagnosis of hemolytic anemia is broad, a systematic approach can allow identification and classification in most cases
- Once the presence of hemolysis is determined, the direct antiglobulin test can diagnose the vast majority of autoimmune hemolytic anemias
- Advanced testing for the diagnosis of the rarer nonimmune acquired hemolytic anemias or hereditary hemolytic anemias should be guided by pretest probability based on the incidence or prevalence and clinical context

INTRODUCTION

The diagnosis, prognosis, and management of autoimmune hemolytic anemia (AIHA) continue to be challenging in clinical practice. Antibodies directed against self-erythrocytes capable of inducing hemolysis at excessive or uncompensated rates result in the entity known as AIHA. These antibodies are usually immunoglobulin G (IgG) in nature, some are capable of fixing complement, and are detected by the direct antiglobulin test (DAT).[1] The DAT is based on specific antibodies to IgG and/or C3d (fragment of the third component of complement) capable of binding to these components on the erythrocyte surface. If the latter molecules are present in sufficient quantity on the erythrocyte membrane, the result is a visible agglutination by cross-linking erythrocytes. In contrast to the DAT, the indirect antiglobulin (indirect Coombs) test is used to detect erythrocyte antibodies in patient serum.

AIHA can be subdivided into warm- or cold-mediated disease based on the optimal thermal amplitude used to detect anti-erythrocyte antibodies. Warm AIHA (WAIHA) is primarily mediated by IgG and hemolysis occurs extravascularly when the IgG heavy

Division of Hematology, Department of Medicine, Mayo Clinic, 200 First Street SW, Rochester, MN 55905, USA
* Corresponding author.
E-mail address: Scheckel.caleb@mayo.edu

Hematol Oncol Clin N Am 36 (2022) 315–324
https://doi.org/10.1016/j.hoc.2021.12.001
0889-8588/22/© 2021 Elsevier Inc. All rights reserved.

chain is recognized by Fc receptors on reticuloendothelial macrophages.[2] In contrast, cold-mediated AIHA, mostly cold agglutinin disease (CAD), is primarily mediated by IgM directed against the I or i antigen. Hemolysis is primarily extravascular and mediated by the complement system due to enhanced opsonization by C3d (some countries outside the United States also report C3b).[3–5]

Primary (idiopathic) AIHA occurs when no disease is clearly associated with the hemolysis, whereas secondary AIHA occurs when hemolytic anemia is directly associated with another disease or drug believed to induce or promote the hemolysis. Primary AIHA comprises ~50% of cases, while secondary AIHA is usually associated with B-cell malignancies, autoimmune diseases, or drugs.[6]

When evaluating a patient with suspected AIHA care must be devoted to using the appropriate methodologies for diagnosis, defining whether AHIA is primary or secondary in type, and consideration of mimicking conditions.[7]

CLINICAL MANIFESTATIONS

Presenting symptoms of AIHA can be heterogenous. Anemia-related symptoms (dyspnea with exertion, fatigue, tachycardia) are present in $3/4$ while jaundice and splenomegaly are only seen in about a third.[8–10] Concurrent immune thrombocytopenia (Evan's syndrome) is only seen in 7%. The severity of symptoms correlates with the degree of anemia, briskness of hemoglobin decline, and underlying comorbidities. Physical examination may reveal pallor, jaundice, tachycardia, or in severe cases, decompensated heart failure. Splenomegaly may be disease-related but can also reflect an underlying lymphoproliferative disorder.[8–10]

INCIDENCE, PREVALENCE, AND DIFFERENTIAL DIAGNOSIS

The incidence of AIHA is considered uncommon, with estimates of 1 to 3 in 1,00,000 population annually.[11] In children and adults, warm-reacting antibodies are the primary pathogenic etiology in most of the cases (~75% and ~90%, respectively).[12,13] The remainder are due to cold-induced or mixed disorders. The incidence of acquired hemolytic anemias is reviewed in **Table 1**.[11,13–18] The prevalence of secondary AIHA in selected conditions is as follows: chronic lymphocytic leukemia 11%, systemic lupus erythematosus (SLE) 10%, allogeneic stem cell transplantation (HCT) 4% to 6%, and non-Hodgkin lymphoma 2% to 3%.[19,20] Secondary AIHA can also be seen with viral infections such as HIV, Epstein Barr virus (EBV), hepatitis C, and SARS-CoV-2.[21,22] Common culprits of drug-induced AIHA include: cephalosporins, penicillin, NSAIDS, sulfa, fludarabine, oxaliplatin, checkpoint inhibitors, and intravenous immunoglobulin.[23] While hereditary hemolytic anemias are more commonly diagnosed during childhood or early adulthood, they can present as symptomatic anemia later in life and should remain in the differential diagnosis during the evaluation of hemolytic anemia. The prevalence of hereditary hemolytic anemias is reviewed in **Table 2**.[24–30]

The DAT remains the cornerstone for the diagnosis of AIHA and enables the distinction between warm forms (70% of cases; DAT positive for IgG or IgG and C), cold agglutinins (20% of cases; DAT positive for C), and mixed forms (<10% of cases, DAT positive for IgG and C, with the coexistence of warm autoantibodies and cold agglutinins). A total of 3% to 11% of patients with hemolytic anemia clinically consistent with WAIHA will have a negative DAT result.[31,32] A negative test result may lead physicians to reject the diagnosis, resulting in additional patient evaluation and delays in treatment. Technical processing is the most common "cause" of DAT-negative WAIHA. Approximately 10% to 50% of patients with DAT-negative WAIHA will have a positive standard DAT result using anti-IgG and anti-C3d reagents retested at

Table 1
Incidence of acquired hemolytic anemias

Type	Disease	Incidence (100,000/y)
Immune	Warm autoimmune	2
	Cold agglutinin disease	0.1
	Paroxysmal cold hemoglobinuria	0.5
	Paroxysmal nocturnal hemoglobinuria	0.1
Microangiopathy	Thrombotic thrombocytopenic purpura	0.3
	Hemolytic uremic syndrome	1
	Atypical hemolytic uremic syndrome	0.2

immunohematology reference laboratories.[31,33,34] If suspicion of WAIHA remains high, DAT should be repeated, preferably by an immunohematology reference laboratory. The presenting clinical features and treatment responses of patients with DAT-negative WAIHA are similar to patients with DAT-positive WAIHA.[35]

Considerations for patients with a positive DAT beyond WAIHA and CAD include alloimmunization, mixed autoimmune hemolytic anemia, and paroxysmal cold hemoglobinuria. A significant transfusion history, a high cold agglutinin titer in the presence of positive DAT, and the Donath–Landsteiner test may clue the clinician in the appropriate direction for each of these conditions, respectively (**Fig. 1**). The DAT results and pattern of antigen involvement may provide clues about the etiology of secondary AIHA (**Fig. 2**).

The differential diagnosis for patients with a negative DAT is more extensive and testing can be guided by the degree of suspicion of a hereditary condition. Clues on history and examination that suggest a hereditary cause of hemolysis include family history, pigmented gallstones, splenomegaly, and chronic anemia. Hemoglobin electrophoresis can establish the diagnosis of various hemoglobinopathies such as sickle cell disease, thalassemia, among others. In patients whereby clinical suspicion of AIHA remains high despite negative DAT, repeat testing with an enhanced DAT may be beneficial.

LABORATORY EVALUATION

Individuals evaluated for AIHA will likely have a CBC as well as other laboratory evidence of hemolysis. The clinical utility of these studies is reviewed later in discussion

Table 2
Prevalence of hereditary hemolytic anemias

Type	Disease	Prevalence Per 100,000 (Patient Race)
Hemoglobinopathy	Sickle cell disease	275 (Black)
	Thalassemia	7
Membranopathy	Hereditary elliptocytosis	25
	Hereditary spherocytosis	20 (White)
	Hereditary stomatocytosis	10
Enzymopathy	G6PD deficiency	10,000 (Black)
	Pyruvate kinase deficiency	5
	Hexokinase deficiency	Unknown
Other	Wilson disease	3

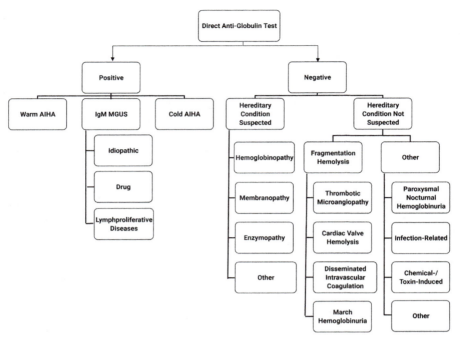

Fig. 1. Evaluation of Hemolysis.

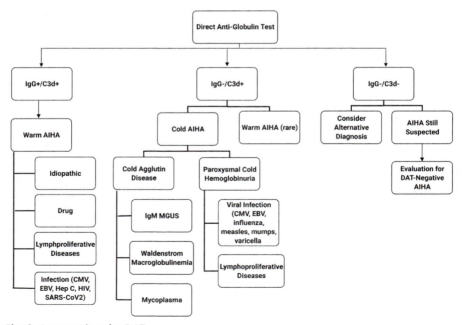

Fig. 2. Interpreting the DAT.

and summarized in **Table 3**. It is important to note that DAT should typically be performed after the presence of hemolysis is determined and not in the reverse order. A positive DAT only means the presence of antibody or complement on the surface of RBCs and is not an evidence of hemolysis. Positive DAT without hemolysis can occur in healthy people (incidental finding) and in certain clinical conditions such as immunoglobulin administration, recent hematopoietic or solid organ transplantation, as well as autoimmune and lymphoproliferative disorders.[36]

Markers of Hemolysis

Typical hemoglobin at presentation is between 7 and 10 g/dL, although values <7 g/dL can be seen in as many as 30%.[8] The anemia is usually normocytic but macrocytosis can be seen due to reticulocytosis. Depending on co-occurring conditions some patients may have leukocytosis (chronic lymphocytic leukemia) or thrombocytopenia (Evan's syndrome). The reticulocyte count increases as the bone marrow increases the production of RBCs to replace those that are lost. The absolute reticulocyte count is the preferred method of measurement because it is unaffected by the hemoglobin concentration. In one series, the mean corrected reticulocyte count was 7.4%.[8] Non-elevated reticulocyte counts can be seen in concomitant conditions that limit RBC production (iron deficiency, underlying bone marrow disorder, drug effect) or

Table 3
Markers of hemolysis

Type	Test	Expected/Comment	Intravascular	Extravascular
Direct	Haptoglobin	Low; most specific	More prominent	Less prominent
	LDH	High; not specific; isoenzyme 1 (RBC and heart)	Less prominent	More prominent
	Indirect bilirubin	High; not specific	Less prominent	More prominent
	AST	High; not specific	Present in both	Present in both
	Blood smear	Variable according to cause: Spherocytes, elliptocytes, schistocytes, sickle cell, etc.	Present in both	Present in both
Indirect	Reticulocyte count	>100 × 10^9/L; normal or low if hypoproliferative component	Present in both	Present in both
	Mean cell volume	High; from reticulocytosis; mostly normal though	Present in both	Present in both
	Soluble transferrin receptor	High (increased RBC turnover); iron deficiency	Present in both	Present in both
	Hemoglobin A1c	Unexpectedly low (limited time for RBC glycation)	Present in both	Present in both
	Carboxyhemoglobin	High (CO a breakdown product of heme metabolism)	Present in both	Present in both

A number of testing abnormalities can be seen in the presence of hemolysis. Direct markers of hemolysis are laboratory abnormalities that correlate to the destruction of RBCs. The degree of abnormality may correlate with the location of hemolysis (ie, intravascular vs extravascular) though the clinical utility is debatable. Indirect markers of hemolysis may act as surrogate markers via reticulocytosis, increased RBC turnover, or heme metabolism.

autoantibodies against RBC precursors.[8,37] The peripheral blood smear may reveal spherocytes and reticulocytes. The absence of certain findings (schistocytes, target cells) can be useful in the differential diagnosis in excluding other conditions.[9,38]

Haptoglobin is commonly low or unmeasurable regardless of whether the hemolytic anemia is primarily intravascular or extravascular. In a series of 100 patients, a haptoglobin less than 25 mg/dL had a sensitivity of 83%, specificity of 96%, and predictive value of 87%.[10,39] Lactate dehydrogenase (LDH) is typically increased with one series reporting a median LDH of approximately 500 units/L.[40] Indirect bilirubin elevations in the range of 2 to 3 mg/dL are common.[41] Aspartate transaminase (AST) is found primarily in the heart, liver, skeletal muscle, red cells, and kidneys.[42] Mild elevations in AST can be seen in hemolysis, though the ratio of LDH/AST is typically over 30.[43] Investigation into AST/ALT ratio as a hemolytic marker in patients with sickle cell disease lacking cardiac or hepatic dysfunction found an inverse relationship between hemoglobin and AST/ALT ratio and positive correlation with reticulocytes and lactate dehydrogenase.[44]

Ferritin can be increased in several chronic hemolytic conditions including enzymopathies, chronic cold agglutinin disease, and congenital dyserythropoietic anemia.[45–47] Ferritin is also an acute-phase protein and increases in various metabolic and inflammatory and the coexistence of these conditions with hemolysis may lead to elevated ferritin values. Longstanding transfusion support may also contribute to iron overload. The soluble transferrin receptor is increased in hemolytic anemia but may also reflect erythropoiesis rather than hemolysis and is also elevated in iron deficiency anemia.[47] Hemosiderinuria is typically associated with marked intravascular hemolysis in excess of haptoglobin binding capacity. It is usually seen 3 to 4 days after the onset of hemolysis and it can persist for several weeks after hemolysis cessation, whereas hemoglobinuria quickly disappears.

Table 4
Evaluation: Hemolysis testing beyond the blood smear

Type	Test	Comment
Autoimmune	Direct antiglobulin (DAT)	Initial test for any type of hemolytic anemia
	Enhanced DAT	DAT negative but AIHA still suspected
	Cold agglutinin titer	Cold agglutinin disease
	Donath–Landsteiner	Paroxysmal cold hemoglobinuria
Other Acquired	ADAMTS13 level	Thrombotic thrombocytopenic purpura
	Serologic complement	Complement-mediated thrombotic microangiopathy
	Genetic complement	Complement-mediated thrombotic microangiopathy
	Flow cytometry	Paroxysmal nocturnal hemoglobinuria
Hereditary	Eosin-5-maleimide (EMA) binding	Hereditary spherocytosis, elliptocytosis (some)
	Osmotic fragility	Hereditary spherocytosis
	RBC enzyme activity	RBC enzymopathy
	Next-generation sequencing	All types; for select patients

When investigating the etiology of hemolysis, a broad differential must be considered. Depending on the clinician's index of suspicion, testing for autoimmune, acquired, or hereditary etiologies may be required.

When interpreting the results of a glycosylated hemoglobin (HbA1c) level, factors affecting the life span of the red blood cells should be kept in mind as they may affect the measurement of the HbA1c. Hemolytic anemia can cause a falsely low HbA1c, thus a patient with diabetes and hemolytic anemia may be falsely considered a well-controlled diabetic. Severe hemolysis can result in an immeasurable HbA1c. Immeasurable HbA1c in a patient with hemolysis may be a marker for potentially fatal hemolysis and thus indicate a poor prognosis.[48,49] Carbon monoxide (CO) is produced endogenously as a byproduct of heme metabolism and carboxyhemoglobin can be elevated during hemolytic anemia. Metabolism of heme via heme oxidase produces one molecule of CO per molecule of heme degraded.[50,51]

Advanced Testing

The focus of additional testing beyond markers of hemolysis and the peripheral blood smear can be guided initially by the clinical and family history, physical examination, presence of other cytopenias, and the results of the DAT. Advanced testing options for when various hemolytic anemias are suspected are summarized in **Table 4**.

SUMMARY

The etiology of AIHA remains incompletely understood; however, the mechanisms of erythrocyte destruction and the clinical complications that accompany this disorder are well defined. Because the causes of hemolytic anemias are numerous, a broad differential diagnosis must be entertained. The clinical heterogeneity of AIHA requires the clinician to clearly define the nature of the disorder for each patient. The need to look for associated diseases is emphasized as their management may aid in AIHA therapy.

CLINICS CARE POINTS

- AIHA may be warm or cold-mediated with either primary or secondary etiologies.
- Presenting symptoms of AIHA can be heterogenous and thorough clinical evaluation may highlight an underlying cause.
- Many potential markers of hemolysis have reasonably high sensitivity but poor specificity.
- DAT should typically be performed after the presence of hemolysis is determined and not in the reverse order.
- The findings on the DAT can guide the differential diagnosis for the AIHA.
- Establishing the diagnosis of AIHA must be accompanied by a thorough evaluation for associated diseases.

REFERENCES

1. Coombs RR, Mourant AE, Race RR. A new test for the detection of weak and incomplete Rh agglutinins. Br J Exp Pathol 1945;26(4):255–66.
2. Brodsky RA. Warm Autoimmune Hemolytic Anemia. N Engl J Med 2019;381:647.
3. Berentsen S. How I manage patients with cold agglutinin disease. Br J Haematol 2018;181:320.
4. Berentsen S, Randen U, Tjønnfjord GE. Cold agglutinin-mediated autoimmune hemolytic anemia. Hematol Oncol Clin North Am 2015;29:455.
5. Swiecicki PL, Hegerova LT, Gertz MA. Cold agglutinin disease. Blood 2013;122:1114.

6. Go RS, Winters JL. Kay NE How I treat autoimmune hemolytic anemia. Blood 2017;129(22):2971–9.

7. Crowther M, Chan YL, Garbett IK, et al. Evidence-based focused review of the treatment of idiopathic warm immune hemolytic anemia in adults. Blood 2011; 118(15):4036–40.

8. Liesveld JL, Rowe JM, Lichtman MA. Variability of the erythropoietic response in autoimmune hemolytic anemia: analysis of 109 cases. Blood 1987;69:820.

9. Roumier M, Loustau V, Guillaud C, et al. Characteristics and outcome of warm autoimmune hemolytic anemia in adults: New insights based on a single-center experience with 60 patients. Am J Hematol 2014;89:E150.

10. Barcellini W, Fattizzo B, Zaninoni A, et al. Clinical heterogeneity and predictors of outcome in primary autoimmune hemolytic anemia: a GIMEMA study of 308 patients. Blood 2014;124:2930.

11. Aladjidi N, Leverger G, Leblanc T, et al. New insights into childhood autoimmune hemolytic anemia: a French national observational study of 265 children. Haematologica 2011;96(5):655–63.

12. Genty I, Michel M, Hermine O, et al. [Characteristics of autoimmune hemolytic anemia in adults: retrospective analysis of 83 cases]. Rev Med Interne 2002; 23(11):901–9.

13. Berentsen S, Ulvestad E, Langholm R, et al. Primary chronic cold agglutinin disease: a population based clinical study of 86 patients. Haematologica 2006; 91(4):460–6.

14. Sokol RJ, Hewitt S, Stamps BK. Autoimmune haemolysis associated with Donath-Landsteiner antibodies. Acta Haematol 1982;68:268–77.

15. Gulbis B, Eleftheriou A, Angastiniotis M, et al. Epidemiology of rare anaemias in Europe. Adv Exp Med Biol 2010;686:375–96.

16. Reese JA, Muthurajah DS, Hovinga JAK, et al. Children and adults with thrombotic thrombocytopenic purpura associated with severe, acquired Adamts13 deficiency: Comparison of incidence, demographic and clinical features. Pediatr Blood Cancer 2013;60:1676–82.

17. Trachtman H, Austin C, Lewinski M, et al. Renal and neurological involvement in typical Shiga toxin-associated HUS. Nat Rev Nephrol 2012;8(11):658–69.

18. Fremeaux-Bacchi V, Fakhouri F, Garnier A, et al. Genetics and Outcome of Atypical Hemolytic Uremic Syndrome: A Nationwide French Series Comparing Child and Adults. Clin J Am Soc Nephrol 2013;8(4):554–62.

19. Barcellini W, Fattizzo B, Zaninoni A. Management of refractory autoimmune hemolytic anemia after allogeneic hematopoietic stem cell transplantation: current perspectives. J Blood Med 2019;10:265.

20. Giannouli S, Voulgarelis M, Ziakas PD, et al. Anaemia in systemic lupus erythematosus: from pathophysiology to clinical assessment. Ann Rheum Dis 2006;65:144.

21. Leaf RK, O'Brien KL, Leaf DE, et al. Autoimmune hemolytic anemia in a young man with acute hepatitis E infection. Am J Hematol 2017;92:E77.

22. Lazarian G, Quinquenel A, Bellal M, et al. Autoimmune haemolytic anaemia associated with COVID-19 infection. Br J Haematol 2020;190:29.

23. Garratty G. Immune hemolytic anemia associated with drug therapy. Blood Rev 2010;24:143–50.

24. Data & Statistics on Sickle Cell Disease. Centers for Disease Control and Prevention. Available at: https://www.cdc.gov/ncbddd/sicklecell/data.html. September 24, 2021.

25. Gallagher PG. Red cell membrane disorders. Hematol Am Soc Hematol Educ Program 2005;13–8.

26. Perrotta S, Gallagher PG, Mohandas N. Hereditary spherocytosis. Lancet 2008; 372(9647):1411–26.
27. King MJ, Garçon L, Hoyer JD, et al, International Council for Standardization in Haematology. ICSH guidelines for the laboratory diagnosis of nonimmune hereditary red cell membrane disorders. Int J Lab Hematol 2015;37(3):304–25.
28. Heller P, Best WR, Nelson RB, et al. Clinical implications of sickle-cell trait and glucose-6-phosphate dehydrogenase deficiency in hospitalized black male patients. N Engl J Med 1979;300:1001–5.
29. Beutler E, Gelbart T. Estimating the prevalence of pyruvate kinase deficiency from the gene frequency in the general white population. Blood 2000;95:3585.
30. Huster D. Wilson disease. Best Pract Res Clin Gastroenterol 2010;24(5):531–9.
31. Segel GB, Lichtman MA. Direct antiglobulin ("Coombs") test-negative autoimmune hemolytic anemia: a review. Blood Cells Mol Dis 2014;52(4):152–60.
32. Karafin MS, Denomme GA, Schanen M, et al. Clinical and reference lab characteristics of patients with suspected direct antiglobulin test (DAT)-negative immune hemolytic anemia. Immunohematology 2015;31(3):108–15.
33. Leger RM, Co A, Hunt P, et al. Attempts to support an immune etiology in 800 patients with direct antiglobulin test-negative hemolytic anemia. Immunohematology 2010;26(4):156–60.
34. Kamesaki T, Toyotsuji T, Kajii E. Characterization of direct antiglobulin test-negative autoimmune hemolytic anemia: a study of 154 cases. Am J Hematol 2013;88(2):93–6.
35. Eaton WW, Rose NR, Kalaydjian A, et al. Epidemiology of autoimmune diseases in Denmark. J Autoimmun 2007;29(1):1–9.
36. Zarandona JM, Yazer MH. The role of the Coombs test in evaluating hemolysis in adults. CMAJ Jan 2006;174(3):305–7.
37. Conley CL, Lippman SM, Ness P. Autoimmune hemolytic anemia with reticulocytopenia. A medical emergency. JAMA 1980;244:1688.
38. Mantripragada K, Quesenberry PJ. Doublet spherocytes. Blood 2014;124:12.
39. Marchand A, Galen RS, Van Lente F. The predictive value of serum haptoglobin in hemolytic disease. JAMA 1980;243:1909.
40. Birgens H, Frederiksen H, Hasselbalch HC, et al. A phase III randomized trial comparing glucocorticoid monotherapy versus glucocorticoid and rituximab in patients with autoimmune haemolytic anaemia. Br J Haematol 2013;163:393.
41. Pratt DS, Kaplan MM. Evaluation of abnormal liver-enzymes results in asymptomatic patients. N Engl J Med 2000;342:1266–71.
42. Omine M. Overview of the clinical reference guides for the idiopathic hematopoietic disorders. Nihon Rinsho Jpn J Clin Med 2008;66(3):433–8.
43. Nsiah K, Dzogbefia VP, Ansong D, et al. Pattern of AST and ALT changes in Relation to Hemolysis in sickle cell Disease. Clin Med Blood Disord 2011. https://doi.org/10.4137/CMBD.S3969.
44. Russo R, Gambale A, Langella C, et al. Retrospective cohort study of 205 cases with congenital dyserythropoietic anemia type II: definition of clinical and molecular spectrum and identification of new diagnostic scores. Am J Hematol 2014; 89(10):E169–75.
45. Mariani M, Barcellini W, Vercellati C, et al. Clinical and hematologic features of 300 patients affected by hereditary spherocytosis grouped according to the type of the membrane protein defect. Haematologica 2008;93(9):1310–7.
46. Zanella A, Fermo E, Bianchi P, et al. Red cell pyruvate kinase deficiency: molecular and clinical aspects. Br J Haematol 2005;130(1):11–25.

47. Kohgo Y, Niitsu Y, Koudo H, et al. Urushizaki I Serum transferrin receptor as a new index of erythropoiesis. Blood 1987;70:1955.

48. Debard A, Charmion S, Ben Ameur S, et al. Inappropriate low glycated hemoglobin and hemolysis. Rev Med Internet 2009;2013:525–7.

49. Jandrić Balen M, Lukenda V, Jandrić I, et al. HbA1C—overall glycemia marker and hemolytic anemia indicator. Med Glas (Zenica) 2012;2013:406–8.

50. Engel RR, Rodkey FL, Krill CE. Carboxyhemoglobin levels as index hemolysis. Pediatr 1971;47:723–30.

51. Hampson NB. Carboxyhemoglobin elevation due to hemolytic anemia. J Emerg Med 2007;33:17–9. https://doi.org/10.1016/j.jemermed.2006.10.004.

Updates in the Management of Warm Autoimmune Hemolytic Anemia

Jennifer C. Yui, MD, MS[a],*, Robert A. Brodsky, MD[b]

KEYWORDS

- Autoimmune hemolytic anemia • Direct antiglobulin test • Immunosuppression
- Hemolysis • Therapy

KEY POINTS

- Autoimmune hemolytic anemia (AIHA) is a heterogeneous disease, with warm-reacting autoantibodies, cold-reacting autoantibodies, or a mixed phenotype of both
- Warm AIHA can either be primary/idiopathic or secondary, typically associated with lymphoproliferative disorders, rheumatologic disease, primary immunodeficiency, or drugs.
- First-line therapy includes glucocorticoids with or without rituximab, with less evidence for the sequence of subsequent therapies such as other immunosuppressive agents or splenectomy
- For relapsed or refractory disease, clinical trials should be offered when available, with investigational agents currently including spleen tyrosine kinase inhibitors; monoclonal antibodies targeting CD38, Bruton's tyrosine kinase inhibitors, complement inhibitors, and antibodies against neonatal Fc receptors.

INTRODUCTION

Autoimmune hemolytic anemia (AIHA) is the destruction of circulating red blood cells (RBCs) secondary to autoantibodies targeting the patient's own RBCs.[1] When RBC destruction is rapid enough that RBC production is unable to compensate, anemia results.

The varied disorders that cause AIHA are divided into warm, cold, or mixed AIHA based on the temperature-dependent activity of the autoantibodies. Warm autoantibodies cause agglutination of the blood at 37°C,[2] cold autoantibodies cause maximal agglutination at 0–4°C,[3] and mixed autoantibodies show activity at both temperatures.[4] Series of consecutive patients have found that 80% to 90% of AIHA in adults[5,6] and 75% of AIHA in children[7] is caused by warm autoantibodies (wAIHA) which are

[a] Division of Hematology, Department of Medicine, Johns Hopkins University School of Medicine, 1830 East Monument Street, Suite 7300, Baltimore, MD 21205, USA; [b] Division of Hematology, Johns Hopkins University School of Medicine, 720 Rutland Ave, Ross Building Rm 1025, Baltimore, MD 21205, USA
* Corresponding author.
E-mail address: jyui1@jhmi.edu

Hematol Oncol Clin N Am 36 (2022) 325–339
https://doi.org/10.1016/j.hoc.2021.11.005
0889-8588/22/© 2021 Elsevier Inc. All rights reserved.

almost always IgG antibodies.[8] wAIHA can be further divided into primary or idiopathic cases, and secondary wAIHA with an associated condition as an identified underlying trigger. These secondary wAIHA comprise 50% of cases,[9] with the treatment of secondary AIHA typically involving the treatment of the underlying disorder, though in severe cases, AIHA-directed therapy may also be required.[10]

EPIDEMIOLOGY

AIHA is a rare disorder, with an incidence of 1 to 3 cases per 100,000 persons annually[9,11] and prevalence of 17 cases per 100,000 persons.[12] There is a slight female predominance, and typical onset is in the fifth decade.[12] For secondary wAIHA, the typical patient characteristics at presentation vary based on the underlying trigger.

Most patients will have a chronic, relapsing disease course, with only approximately 30% historically achieving a durable remission with initial therapy only.[13,14]

PATHOPHYSIOLOGY

The auto-antibodies in wAIHA are panagglutinins, directed at antigens which are present on RBCs in nearly all individuals, often proteins on the Rh complex,[15,16] and glycophorin antigens on the RBC membrane.[17] Warm antibodies are nearly universally polyclonal, even when secondary to clonal processes such as hematologic malignancies.[18]

The mechanism of anemia in wAIHA is multifactorial, involving extracellular hemolysis with clearance of IgG-coated RBCs by splenic macrophages, antibody-dependent cell-mediated cytotoxicity, and complement activation. These splenic macrophages have Fc gamma receptors for IgG heavy chains, which recognize the IgG-coated RBCs and phagocytose the IgG heavy chain and a portion of the membrane.[19] When the RBC membrane reseals, the resultant RBC, termed a spherocyte/microspherocyte, has a reduced surface-to-volume ratio. These spherocytes have poor deformability and become trapped in the splenic sinusoids, leading to phagocytic clearance. CD8+ T cells and natural killer cells in the spleen may also cause extracellular hemolysis via antibody-dependent cell-mediated cytotoxicity.

Complement deposition leads to extravascular hemolysis through opsonization.[20] In severe cases, complement deposition may also cause membrane attack complex formation on the surface of RBCs and subsequent intravascular hemolysis.[21]

The processes that lead to autoantibody generation are complex and not fully understood, but include immune dysregulation and breakdown of immune self-tolerance.[19] Molecular mimicry of foreign antigens from exogenous exposures such as viral infections and drugs can lead to cross-reactivity with endogenous RBC antigens.[22] Altered T cell function and T-helper subsets have a critical role in the loss of self-tolerance, as normal regulatory processes include the apoptosis of autoreactive T cell clones.

Secondary Warm Autoimmune Hemolytic Anemia

Roughly 50% of wAIHA has an associated underlying condition, often with a component of immune activation, dysregulation, or deficiency. The most common causes of secondary wAIHA are malignancy, immunodeficiency, autoimmune disease, infection, and medications.[6,23]

Acquired lymphoproliferative disorders, including chronic lymphocytic leukemia (CLL)[18] and non-Hodgkin lymphoma[24,25] are among the most common causes of wAIHA, and the diagnosis of wAIHA may precede the diagnosis of malignancy by years.[26] There is also a high prevalence of monoclonal gammopathy in patients with wAIHA,[27] though pathogenicity of the monoclonal protein has not been established.

The most common lymphoproliferative disorder associated with wAIHA is CLL, with 4% to 10% of patients with CLL developing wAIHA.[18,28] In patients with CLL, the antibody is not directly produced by the clonal cells, but by nonmalignant B cells.[29] wAIHA is not an adverse prognostic indicator in CLL.[30] The incidence of AIHA in CLL is increased when patients are treated with purine analogs such as fludarabine,[31,32] pentostatin,[33] or cladribine,[34] but not with alkylating agents[35] or newer agents such as ibrutinib.[36]

Immunodeficiency disorders are also implicated in secondary wAIHA, including common variable immunodeficiency[37] and autoimmune lymphoproliferative syndrome (ALPS).[38] Patients with ALPS have mutations causing defects in Fas-mediated apoptosis, which allow for the survival of autoreactive lymphocytes. In a series of 265 children with AIHA, 15% were found to have a primary immunodeficiency.[7] All pediatric patients and young adults presenting with wAIHA should have an immunologic evaluation performed to screen for these conditions.[39]

In patients who have undergone allogeneic stem cell transplantation, antibodies directed at recipient RBCs may cause wAIHA.[40,41] Recipients of solid organ transplants may develop wAIHA due to passenger lymphocyte syndrome, in which donor-derived lymphocytes are transferred along with the organ allograft, and lead to antibody production against recipient RBCs.[42,43]

wAIHA occurs frequently in patients with other autoimmune diseases,[39] most commonly systemic lupus erythematosus.[44]

Infections, particularly viral infections,[45,46] have been implicated in the development of wAIHA. Human immunodeficiency virus infection leads to immune dysregulation which can result in wAIHA.[47] Babesiosis may cause wAIHA, particularly in asplenic patients.[48] Recently, wAIHA has also been described in the setting of COVID-19 infection.[49,50]

More than 150 medications can trigger AIHA, with drug-induced AIHA comprising 10% of all AIHA[5,51] Common causal medications[52–54] include cephalosporins, penicillins, beta-lactamase inhibitors, NSAIDs, quinine, lorazepam, quinine, and more recently checkpoint inhibitors[55] with wAIHA occurring more frequently with PD-1 and PD-L1 inhibitors (0.15%–0.25%) than CTLA-4 inhibitors (0.06%).

Primary mechanisms of drug-induced AIHA include a hapten (penicillin type) reaction in which autoantibody binds drug which is firmly bound to the RBC membrane without complement activation and immune complex (ternary complex) reaction for which the drug is loosely bound to the RBC membrane and activates complement, often causing a more severe hemolysis.[56–58] In the case of checkpoint inhibitors, the mechanism is thought to be immune dysregulation and redirected immune surveillance, so these patients often do not respond to drug cessation alone.[55]

CLINICAL PRESENTATION

The severity of the symptoms on presentation is proportional to the degree of anemia. Brisk hemolysis may cause severe, life-threatening anemia. Common presenting symptoms include fatigue, generalized weakness, and dyspnea on exertion. Depending on the degree of hemolysis, physical examination may reveal pallor, jaundice, and splenomegaly.

Laboratory features include low hemoglobin, reticulocytosis, and elevated lactate dehydrogenase. While the hemolysis associated with wAIHA is extravascular, there is often a component of intravascular hemolysis,[9] with low haptoglobin and indirect hyperbilirubinemia. In a series of 109 cases of hemolytic anemia, the mean hematocrit at presentation was 24% with mean corrected reticulocyte percentage of 5%.[59]

While wAIHA typically presents with isolated anemia, it may present concomitantly or sequentially with immune thrombocytopenia and with immune neutropenia, as Evans syndrome.[60]

In patients with the above markers of hemolytic anemia, the peripheral blood smear and direct antiglobulin test (DAT) should be performed to further characterize the hemolytic anemia. The peripheral blood smear in wAIHA often demonstrates microspherocytes (**Fig. 1**). Other peripheral blood smear findings may include polychromasia and Howell Jolly bodies in asplenic patients.

The DAT, or Coombs test, is used to detect the presence of IgG and/or complement on patient RBCs. The DAT relies on a polyspecific anti-human globulin which causes agglutination of antibody-coated RBCs.[61] Patient RBCs are washed and then incubated with anti-human IgG antibodies, causing agglutination of IgG-coated RBCs. The washed RBCs are also incubated with anti-human C3d antibodies to detect complement.

The indirect antiglobulin test detects unbound antibodies in patient eluate.[8] This method can distinguish autoantibodies from alloantibodies, as alloantibodies will only react with donor RBCs with a specific antigen, whereas most autoantibodies are panagglutinins that react with all donor RBCs.[9]

In wAIHA, the DAT typically demonstrates agglutination with anti-IgG, with or without agglutination with anti-C3.[62] Cold agglutinin disease is typically caused by IgM antibodies which react at low temperatures, causing complement-mediated hemolysis, so the DAT is negative for IgG but positive for C3.[63] Patients may also present with a mixed phenotype with both a warm- and cold-reactive antibodies.[4]

Rarely (<5% of cases), wAIHA can present with negative DAT, typically due to low-affinity IgG autoantibodies affected by the preparative washes, or antibody below the level of detection of commercial anti-IgG reagents, or because the pathogenic autoantibodies are IgA antibodies or monomeric or warm-reacting IgM antibodies.[64] In these cases, diagnosis may be aided by enhanced DAT methods, with which 31% to 55% of patients with DAT-negative wAIHA will have a positive result.[65,66]

The DAT may be positive in up to 8% of hospitalized patients with no clinical evidence of hemolysis.[67] In the acute setting, a positive DAT may occur with delayed hemolytic transfusions reactions[68] or after therapies such as intravenous immunoglobulin (IVIG)[69] or daratumumab.[70] Given these test characteristics, the diagnosis of wAIHA should be based on DAT results and clinical evidence of hemolysis.

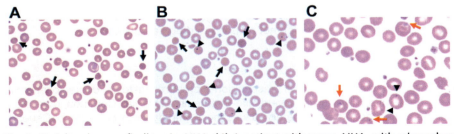

Fig. 1. Peripheral smear findings in AIHA. (*A*) A patient with warm AIHA, with microspherocytes (*black arrows*). (*B*) Postsplenectomy patient with warm AIHA, with microspherocytes (*black arrows*) and Howell Jolly bodies (*black arrow heads*). (*C*) Postsplenectomy patient with AIHA secondary to babesiosis infection with intracellular forms (*red arrows*) and Howell Jolly bodies (*black arrow heads*).

In patients with wAIHA, evaluation for secondary causes should be part of the initial evaluation. A single-institution series demonstrated that greater than 50% of secondary wAIHA can be caused by underlying lymphoproliferative disorder.[59] Peripheral blood flow cytometry should be obtained in all patients with wAIHA,[1] with the consideration of imaging and bone marrow biopsy in patients with constitutional symptoms or lymphadenopathy.[71] In patients with signs and symptoms of rheumatologic disease, appropriate serologic testing should be performed.

Patients with wAIHA may also present with thrombotic complications, which often occur early in the clinical presentation.[14] Thrombotic risk is increased in the setting of inflammation-causing endothelial dysfunction, and free hemoglobin from the lysed RBCs decreasing serum nitric oxide, allowing for increased platelet aggregation.[72,73] Given the high incidence of VTE, clinicians should maintain a high index of suspicion for VTE, obtaining diagnostic imaging in patients with consistent signs or symptoms including dyspnea out of proportion to the degree of anemia. We consider thromboses in the setting of active AIHA to be provoked events, and it is reasonable to discontinue anticoagulation (in the absence of ongoing risk factor for VTE) after a limited course of anticoagulation if there is no evidence of active hemolysis.

TREATMENT
Transfusion

Hemolytic crises may occur with severe anemia (hemoglobin < 6 g/dL) causing hemodynamic instability and should be treated as a medical emergency. A series of 44 patients with severe wAIHA requiring intensive care reported 30% mortality.[74] These patients should receive transfusion as their initial therapy. Standard cross-matching generally will not yield any compatible blood, given that the pan-reactive antibodies will react with virtually all donor RBCs.[8] While the autoantibodies may also lead to hemolysis of the transfused blood in vivo, transfusion should not be withheld for this reason.[75]

Special procedures are necessary for proper cross-matching, which involve adsorbing the autoantibody with either autologous RBCs or selected donor RBCs and then performing cross-matching using this adsorbed serum.[71] Patients should receive ABO- and RhD-matched blood, with extended phenotype matching as available, pending the urgency of transfusion and risk of alloimmunization.[75] Even in patients at higher risk of alloimmunization, such as patients with a history of prior blood transfusion or pregnancy, benefits of transfusion outweigh the risks.[76] Blood should be transfused at a slow rate, particularly for those at higher risk of sensitization.[77]

First-Line Treatment

Fig. 2 provides a treatment algorithm for wAIHA. Glucocorticoids are the cornerstone of pharmacologic treatment of wAIHA, with mechanisms including decreased antibody production, suppression of phagocytosis by macrophages, and decreased autoantibody affinity to RBCs.[78] Still, there is limited evidence driving optimal dosing and taper schedule.[39,71] Per expert consensus, steroids should be started at a dose of prednisone 1 to 1.5 mg/kg daily or an equivalent dose of IV methylprednisolone.[79,80] The initial dose is continued for at least 2 weeks, before tapering, and a higher rate of relapse occurs when steroids are tapered rapidly over the course of 3 to 4 weeks.[1,51] In more severe presentations of wAIHA or for cases of Evans syndrome, case reports have described administering methylprednisolone 250 to 1000 mg/d for the first 1 to 3 days,[81,82] although there is no data comparing these different dosing strategies.

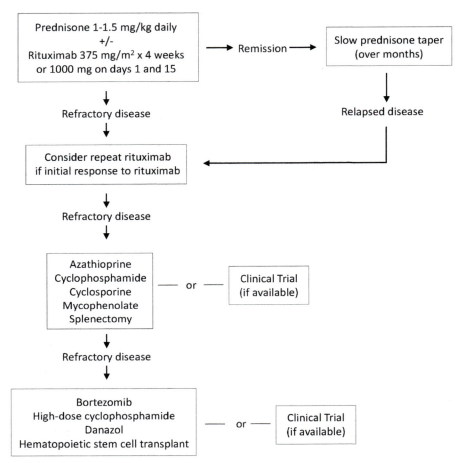

Fig. 2. Treatment algorithm.

The response rate to glucocorticoids is 80% to 90%,[13,14] but only 20% to 30% achieve a durable remission with single-agent glucocorticoids.[14,59] Increased severity of anemia at presentation has been correlated with increased risk of relapse and requiring multiple lines of therapy.[14]

Alternatively, first-line therapy increasingly has included treatment with both glucocorticoids and rituximab, a monoclonal antibody directed at CD20 expressed on B lymphocytes.[83] In one phase 3 trial of 64 patients with wAIHA randomized either to prednisolone alone or prednisolone with rituximab 375 mg/m^2 for 4 weekly doses, the addition of rituximab had superior relapse-free survival at 36 months of follow-up (70% vs 45%).[84] In another randomized trial, 32 patients with wAIHA received either prednisone alone or prednisone with rituximab 1000 mg on days 1 and 15. The addition of rituximab was associated with higher rate of remission at 1 year (75% vs 31%) and 2 years of follow-up (63% vs 19%).[85] The 2-year overall survival in this study was also higher in those who received rituximab (100% vs 63%), though this study was not powered to study survival. In both studies, there was not an increase in adverse effects with the addition of rituximab. A meta-analysis of 21 observational studies of 409 patients with AIHA, of which 183 had wAIHA, found that rituximab was well-tolerated, with mild to moderate adverse events including infusion-related side effects.[86] In the patients with wAIHA, the overall response rate was 70%, with complete response rate 40%. However, data are generally lacking on whether the addition of rituximab leads to improved long-term remission, and more than 30% of patients may relapse in 3 years.[86,87] Of patients with relapsed disease, most will achieve a second remission after a repeat course of rituximab.[59,88,89]

Relapsed and Refractory Disease

Refractory disease is likely if there is no response to glucocorticoids after 21 days.[39] Go and colleagues[71] provide 3 scenarios that would prompt a subsequent line of therapy: (1) requiring the equivalent of prednisone 20 mg daily or more to control hemolysis, (2) clinically significant relapse with hemoglobin less than 11 g/dL or symptomatic hemolytic anemia, and (3) intolerance of a currently effective treatment.

The First International Consensus Meeting's 2020 recommendations provided definitions for complete response and response, which may help standardize future therapy studies: complete response is defined as the normalization of hemoglobin, no evidence of hemolysis (normal bilirubin, LDH, haptoglobin, and reticulocytes), and transfusion independence. Response is defined as an increase in hemoglobin by > 2 g/dL or normalization of hemoglobin without biochemical resolution of hemolysis; and absence of transfusion for the last 7 days.[39]

Historically, splenectomy has been the treatment of choice for patients with relapsed and refractory disease, with a response rate more than 50% in this setting.[90–92] Evidence on the durability of remission is limited,[1] though one study of 15 patients with wAIHA and splenectomy demonstrated a 90% complete response rate and 30% relapse rate at 4.5 years follow-up,[92] and another study of 26 splenectomized patients had a 75% response rate and 30% relapse rate at median follow-up of 41 months.[14] Major risks associated with splenectomy include infection, a risk not fully mitigated by vaccination and antibiotic prophylaxis,[79] and thrombotic complications, described as occurring in nearly 25% of patients postsplenectomy.[14] Thus, use of splenectomy has declined over time, with many favoring rituximab in patients who did not receive upfront rituximab, or who had an initial response to rituximab.[79,93] In the meta-analysis of 21 studies, the overall response rate of rituximab in relapsed or refractory wAIHA was 79%.[86]

Other immunosuppressive therapies have been described for use in relapsed or refractory wAIHA, though evidence is limited to case reports and small series. These agents include azathioprine,[94,95] cyclophosphamide,[94] cyclosporine,[96] and mycophenolate mofetil.[97] Severe refractory wAIHA has been treated with high dose cyclophosphamide.[98] Prospective randomized controlled trials comparing these treatments are lacking, so the appropriate sequence of treatments, including the optimal timing of potential splenectomy, is unclear.[79,80] Patients who do not respond to one immunosuppressive agent may respond to another, so the goal is maximizing safety and controlling hemolysis, given that most patients have chronic disease.[1] Other therapies include the oral androgen danazol,[99] proteasome inhibition with bortezomib,[100] and hematopoietic stem cell transplant in select cases.[101] Sirolimus has been effective particularly in pediatric patients with ALPS.[102]

Investigational Agents

When available, clinical trials should be offered[39] **Fig. 3** demonstrates targeted treatments for wAIHA that are either currently being studied in clinical trials for the treatment of wAIHA, or that have been described in case reports. The targeted

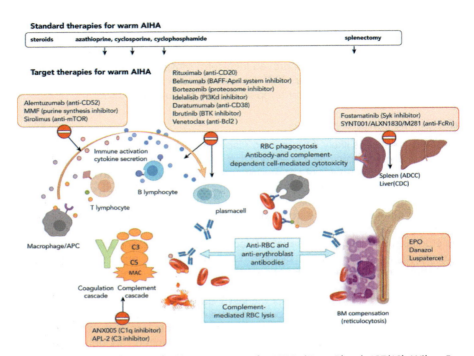

Fig. 3. Investigational agents for the treatment of wAIHA. (*From* Blood, 137(10), Wilma Barcellini and Bruno Fattizzo, "How I treat Warm Autoimmune Hemolytic Anemia," 1283 to 1294, Copyright American Society of Hematology (2021).)

immunologic mechanisms are indicated. None of the targeted therapies depicted are FDA approved for the treatment of wAIHA.[79]

The spleen tyrosine kinase inhibitor fostamatinib,[103] currently used for the treatment of immune thrombocytopenia, has been studied in an open-label phase 2 study,[104] and is being studied in a phase 3 randomized controlled trial.[105] Daratumumab, a monoclonal antibody targeting CD38 has been used in the treatment of cases of AIHA in the setting of HSCT,[106,107] with further investigations underway.[108] The Bruton's tyrosine kinase inhibitor ibrutinib has been used to treat AIHA with underlying CLL,[109,110] with further study underway for AIHA outside of the setting of underlying CLL.[111,112]

Additional investigational treatments include complement inhibitors[113] and antibodies to neonatal Fc receptors.[114–116]

SUMMARY

Warm autoimmune hemolytic anemia (wAIHA) is an uncommon and heterogeneous disorder caused by autoantibodies to RBC antigens. Initial evaluation should involve the DAT, with wAIHA typically IgG positive with or without C3 positivity, and a search for underlying conditions associated with secondary wAIHA, which comprise 50% of cases. First-line therapy involves glucocorticoids, increasingly with rituximab, though a chronic, relapsing course is typical. While a number of immunosuppressive therapies and splenectomy have been used in the setting of relapsed and refractory disease, further study is necessary to determine the optimal choice and sequence of therapies. For relapsed or refractory disease, clinical trials should be offered when available, with investigational agents currently including spleen tyrosine kinase inhibitors, monoclonal antibodies targeting CD38, Bruton's tyrosine kinase inhibitors, complement inhibitors, and antibodies against neonatal Fc receptors.

CLINICS CARE POINTS

- Diagnosis of wAIHA should be based on evidence of hemolysis and DAT results.
- Initial evaluation should also include evaluation for potential causes of secondary wAIHA including lymphoproliferative disease, rheumatologic disease, infection, and causal drugs.
- Initial therapy consists of glucocorticoids, increasingly with concomitant rituximab given superior response, though the durability of response is not well known.
- Many options for subsequent therapies have been described, including splenectomy and immunosuppressive agents, but data on the optimal sequence and dosing are lacking, and clinical trials should be offered when available.

DISCLOSURE

R.A. Brodsky has served on the scientific advisory board for Alexion and has received royalties for authoring chapters for UpToDate.

REFERENCES

1. Brodsky RA. Warm Autoimmune Hemolytic Anemia. N Engl J Med 2019;381(7): 647–54.
2. Stahl D, Sibrowski W. Warm autoimmune hemolytic anemia is an IgM-IgG immune complex disease. J Autoimmun 2005;25(4):272–82.
3. Gertz MA. Cold agglutinin disease. Haematologica 2006;91(4):439–41.
4. Shulman IA, Branch DR, Nelson JM, et al. Autoimmune hemolytic anemia with both cold and warm autoantibodies. JAMA 1985;253(12):1746–8.
5. Liesveld JL, Rowe JM, Lichtman MA. Variability of the erythropoietic response in autoimmune hemolytic anemia: analysis of 109 cases. Blood 1987;69(3):820–6.
6. Genty I, Michel M, Hermine O, et al. [Characteristics of autoimmune hemolytic anemia in adults: retrospective analysis of 83 cases]. Rev Med Interne 2002; 23(11):901–9.
7. Aladjidi N, Leverger G, Leblanc T, et al. New insights into childhood autoimmune hemolytic anemia: a French national observational study of 265 children. Haematologica 2011;96(5):655–63.
8. Packman CH. Hemolytic anemia due to warm autoantibodies. Blood Rev 2008; 22(1):17–31.
9. Gehrs BC, Friedberg RC. Autoimmune hemolytic anemia. Am J Hematol 2002; 69(4):258–71.
10. Hill QA, Stamps R, Massey E, et al. Guidelines on the management of drug-induced immune and secondary autoimmune, haemolytic anaemia. Br J Haematol 2017;177(2):208–20.
11. Klein NP, Ray P, Carpenter D, et al. Rates of autoimmune diseases in Kaiser Permanente for use in vaccine adverse event safety studies. Vaccine 2010;28(4):1062–8.
12. Eaton WW, Rose NR, Kalaydjian A, et al. Epidemiology of autoimmune diseases in Denmark. J Autoimmun 2007;29(1):1–9.
13. Allgood JW, Chaplin H Jr. Idiopathic acquired autoimmune hemolytic anemia. A review of forty-seven cases treated from 1955 through 1965. Am J Med 1967; 43(2):254–73.

14. Barcellini W, Fattizzo B, Zaninoni A, et al. Clinical heterogeneity and predictors of outcome in primary autoimmune hemolytic anemia: a GIMEMA study of 308 patients. Blood 2014;124(19):2930–6.

15. Barker RN, Hall AM, Standen GR, et al. Identification of T-cell epitopes on the Rhesus polypeptides in autoimmune hemolytic anemia. Blood 1997;90(7): 2701–15.

16. Zupanska B, Sokol RJ, Booker DJ, et al. Erythrocyte autoantibodies, the monocyte monolayer assay and in vivo haemolysis. Br J Haematol 1993;84(1): 144–50.

17. Garratty G, Arndt P, Domen R, et al. Severe autoimmune hemolytic anemia associated with IgM warm autoantibodies directed against determinants on or associated with glycophorin A. Vox Sang 1997;72(2):124–30.

18. Mauro FR, Foa R, Cerretti R, et al. Autoimmune hemolytic anemia in chronic lymphocytic leukemia: clinical, therapeutic, and prognostic features. Blood 2000; 95(9):2786–92.

19. Barcellini W. New Insights in the Pathogenesis of Autoimmune Hemolytic Anemia. Transfus Med Hemother 2015;42(5):287–93.

20. Brodsky RA. Complement in hemolytic anemia. Blood 2015;126(22):2459–65.

21. McCann EL, Shirey RS, Kickler TS, et al. IgM autoagglutinins in warm autoimmune hemolytic anemia: a poor prognostic feature. Acta Haematol 1992; 88(2–3):120–5.

22. Barros MM, Blajchman MA, Bordin JO. Warm autoimmune hemolytic anemia: recent progress in understanding the immunobiology and the treatment. Transfus Med Rev 2010;24(3):195–210.

23. Bass GF, Tuscano ET, Tuscano JM. Diagnosis and classification of autoimmune hemolytic anemia. Autoimmun Rev 2014;13(4–5):560–4.

24. Fallah M, Liu X, Ji J, et al. Autoimmune diseases associated with non-Hodgkin lymphoma: a nationwide cohort study. Ann Oncol 2014;25(10):2025–30.

25. Sallah S, Sigounas G, Vos P, et al. Autoimmune hemolytic anemia in patients with non-Hodgkin's lymphoma: characteristics and significance. Ann Oncol 2000; 11(12):1571–7.

26. Rottenberg Y, Yahalom V, Shinar E, et al. Blood donors with positive direct antiglobulin tests are at increased risk for cancer. Transfusion 2009;49(5):838–42.

27. Ravindran A, Sankaran J, Jacob EK, et al. High prevalence of monoclonal gammopathy among patients with warm autoimmune hemolytic anemia. Am J Hematol 2017;92(8):E164–6.

28. De Rossi G, Granati L, Girelli G, et al. Incidence and prognostic significance of autoantibodies against erythrocytes and platelets in chronic lymphocytic leukemia (CLL). Nouv Rev Fr Hematol 1988;30(5–6):403–6.

29. Efremov DG, Ivanovski M, Siljanovski N, et al. Restricted immunoglobulin VH region repertoire in chronic lymphocytic leukemia patients with autoimmune hemolytic anemia. Blood 1996;87(9):3869–76.

30. Ricci F, Tedeschi A, Vismara E, et al. Should a positive direct antiglobulin test be considered a prognostic predictor in chronic lymphocytic leukemia? Clin Lymphoma Myeloma Leuk 2013;13(4):441–6.

31. Gonzalez H, Leblond V, Azar N, et al. Severe autoimmune hemolytic anemia in eight patients treated with fludarabine. Hematol Cell Ther 1998;40(3):113–8.

32. Myint H, Copplestone JA, Orchard J, et al. Fludarabine-related autoimmune haemolytic anaemia in patients with chronic lymphocytic leukaemia. Br J Haematol 1995;91(2):341–4.

33. Byrd JC, Hertler AA, Weiss RB, et al. Fatal recurrence of autoimmune hemolytic anemia following pentostatin therapy in a patient with a history of fludarabine-associated hemolytic anemia. Ann Oncol 1995;6(3):300–1.
34. Fleischman RA, Croy D. Acute onset of severe autoimmune hemolytic anemia after treatment with 2-chlorodeoxyadenosine for chronic lymphocytic leukemia. Am J Hematol 1995;48(4):293.
35. Laurenti L, Autore F, Innocenti I, et al. Autoimmune hemolytic anemia during bendamustine plus rituximab treatment in CLL patients: multicenter experience. Leuk Lymphoma 2016;57(10):2429–31.
36. Burger JA, Tedeschi A, Barr PM, et al. Ibrutinib as Initial Therapy for Patients with Chronic Lymphocytic Leukemia. N Engl J Med 2015;373(25):2425–37.
37. Podjasek JC, Abraham RS. Autoimmune cytopenias in common variable immunodeficiency. Front Immunol 2012;3:189.
38. Straus SE, Sneller M, Lenardo MJ, et al. An inherited disorder of lymphocyte apoptosis: the autoimmune lymphoproliferative syndrome. Ann Intern Med 1999;130(7):591–601.
39. Jager U, Barcellini W, Broome CM, et al. Diagnosis and treatment of autoimmune hemolytic anemia in adults: Recommendations from the First International Consensus Meeting. Blood Rev 2020;41:100648.
40. Sokol RJ, Stamps R, Booker DJ, et al. Posttransplant immune-mediated hemolysis. Transfusion 2002;42(2):198–204.
41. Hows J, Beddow K, Gordon-Smith E, et al. Donor-derived red blood cell antibodies and immune hemolysis after allogeneic bone marrow transplantation. Blood 1986;67(1):177–81.
42. Yazer MH, Triulzi DJ. Immune hemolysis following ABO-mismatched stem cell or solid organ transplantation. Curr Opin Hematol 2007;14(6):664–70.
43. Audet M, Panaro F, Piardi T, et al. Passenger lymphocyte syndrome and liver transplantation. Clin Dev Immunol 2008;2008:715769.
44. Jeffries M, Hamadeh F, Aberle T, et al. Haemolytic anaemia in a multi-ethnic cohort of lupus patients: a clinical and serological perspective. Lupus 2008; 17(8):739–43.
45. Buchanan GR, Boxer LA, Nathan DG. The acute and transient nature of idiopathic immune hemolytic anemia in childhood. J Pediatr 1976;88(5):780–3.
46. Zupanska B, Lawkowicz W, Gorska B, et al. Autoimmune haemolytic anaemia in children. Br J Haematol 1976;34(3):511–20.
47. De Angelis V, Biasinutto C, Pradella P, et al. Clinical significance of positive direct antiglobulin test in patients with HIV infection. Infection 1994;22(2):92–5.
48. Woolley AE, Montgomery MW, Savage WJ, et al. Post-Babesiosis Warm Autoimmune Hemolytic Anemia. N Engl J Med 2017;376(10):939–46.
49. Lazarian G, Quinquenel A, Bellal M, et al. Autoimmune haemolytic anaemia associated with COVID-19 infection. Br J Haematol 2020;190(1):29–31.
50. Lopez C, Kim J, Pandey A, et al. Simultaneous onset of COVID-19 and autoimmune haemolytic anaemia. Br J Haematol 2020;190(1):31–2.
51. Petz LG G. Immune hemolytic anemias. 2nd Edition. Philadelphia, (PA): Churchill Livingstone; 2003.
52. Johnson ST, Fueger JT, Gottschall JL. One center's experience: the serology and drugs associated with drug-induced immune hemolytic anemia–a new paradigm. Transfusion 2007;47(4):697–702.
53. Garbe E, Andersohn F, Bronder E, et al. Drug induced immune haemolytic anaemia in the Berlin Case-Control Surveillance Study. Br J Haematol 2011; 154(5):644–53.

54. Mayer B, Bartolmas T, Yurek S, et al. Variability of Findings in Drug-Induced Immune Haemolytic Anaemia: Experience over 20 Years in a Single Centre. Transfus Med Hemother 2015;42(5):333–9.
55. Tanios GE, Doley PB, Munker R. Autoimmune hemolytic anemia associated with the use of immune checkpoint inhibitors for cancer: 68 cases from the Food and Drug Administration database and review. Eur J Haematol 2019;102(2):157–62.
56. Harris JW. Studies on the mechanism of a drug-induced hemolytic anemia. J Lab Clin Med 1956;47(5):760–75.
57. Salama A, Mueller-Eckhardt C. On the mechanisms of sensitization and attachment of antibodies to RBC in drug-induced immune hemolytic anemia. Blood 1987;69(4):1006–10.
58. Salama A, Santoso S, Mueller-Eckhardt C. Antigenic determinants responsible for the reactions of drug-dependent antibodies with blood cells. Br J Haematol 1991;78(4):535–9.
59. Roumier M, Loustau V, Guillaud C, et al. Characteristics and outcome of warm autoimmune hemolytic anemia in adults: New insights based on a single-center experience with 60 patients. Am J Hematol 2014;89(9):E150–5.
60. Evans RS, Takahashi K, Duane RT, et al. Primary thrombocytopenic purpura and acquired hemolytic anemia; evidence for a common etiology. AMA Arch Intern Med 1951;87(1):48–65.
61. Zantek ND, Koepsell SA, Tharp DR Jr, et al. The direct antiglobulin test: a critical step in the evaluation of hemolysis. Am J Hematol 2012;87(7):707–9.
62. Wheeler CA, Calhoun L, Blackall DP. Warm reactive autoantibodies: clinical and serologic correlations. Am J Clin Pathol 2004;122(5):680–5.
63. Berentsen S. Complement Activation and Inhibition in Autoimmune Hemolytic Anemia: Focus on Cold Agglutinin Disease. Semin Hematol 2018;55(3):141–9.
64. Segel GB, Lichtman MA. Direct antiglobulin ("Coombs") test-negative autoimmune hemolytic anemia: a review. Blood Cells Mol Dis 2014;52(4):152–60.
65. Leger RM, Co A, Hunt P, et al. Attempts to support an immune etiology in 800 patients with direct antiglobulin test-negative hemolytic anemia. Immunohematology 2010;26(4):156–60.
66. Karafin MS, Denomme GA, Schanen M, et al. Clinical and reference lab characteristics of patients with suspected direct antiglobulin test (DAT)-negative immune hemolytic anemia. Immunohematology 2015;31(3):108–15.
67. Meulenbroek EM, Wouters D, Zeerleder SS. Lyse or not to lyse: Clinical significance of red blood cell autoantibodies. Blood Rev 2015;29(6):369–76.
68. Toy PT, Chin CA, Reid ME, et al. Factors associated with positive direct antiglobulin tests in pretransfusion patients: a case-control study. Vox Sang 1985;49(3):215–20.
69. Robertson VM, Dickson LG, Romond EH, et al. Positive antiglobulin tests due to intravenous immunoglobulin in patients who received bone marrow transplant. Transfusion 1987;27(1):28–31.
70. Chapuy CI, Nicholson RT, Aguad MD, et al. Resolving the daratumumab interference with blood compatibility testing. Transfusion 2015;55(6 Pt 2):1545–54.
71. Go RS, Winters JL, Kay NE. How I treat autoimmune hemolytic anemia. Blood 2017;129(22):2971–9.
72. Ataga KI. Hypercoagulability and thrombotic complications in hemolytic anemias. Haematologica 2009;94(11):1481–4.
73. Cappellini MD. Coagulation in the pathophysiology of hemolytic anemias. Hematol Am Soc Hematol Educ Program 2007;74–8.

74. Lafarge A, Bertinchamp R, Pichereau C, et al. Prognosis of autoimmune hemo-lytic anemia in critically ill patients. Ann Hematol 2019;98(3):589–94.
75. Naik R. Warm autoimmune hemolytic anemia. Hematol Oncol Clin North Am 2015;29(3):445–53.
76. Yurek S, Mayer B, Almahallawi M, et al. Precautions surrounding blood transfu-sion in autoimmune haemolytic anaemias are overestimated. Blood Transfus 2015;13(4):616–21.
77. Lechner K, Jager U. How I treat autoimmune hemolytic anemias in adults. Blood 2010;116(11):1831–8.
78. King KE, Ness PM. Treatment of autoimmune hemolytic anemia. Semin Hematol 2005;42(3):131–6.
79. Barcellini W, Fattizzo B. How I treat warm autoimmune hemolytic anemia. Blood 2021;137(10):1283–94.
80. Crowther M, Chan YL, Garbett IK, et al. Evidence-based focused review of the treatment of idiopathic warm immune hemolytic anemia in adults. Blood 2011; 118(15):4036–40.
81. Meyer O, Stahl D, Beckhove P, et al. Pulsed high-dose dexamethasone in chronic autoimmune haemolytic anaemia of warm type. Br J Haematol 1997; 98(4):860–2.
82. Ozsoylu F. Megadose methylprednisolone for the treatment of patients with Evans syndrome. Pediatr Hematol Oncol 2004;21(8):739–40.
83. Dierickx D, Kentos A, Delannoy A. The role of rituximab in adults with warm anti-body autoimmune hemolytic anemia. Blood 2015;125(21):3223–9.
84. Birgens H, Frederiksen H, Hasselbalch HC, et al. A phase III randomized trial comparing glucocorticoid monotherapy versus glucocorticoid and rituximab in patients with autoimmune haemolytic anaemia. Br J Haematol 2013;163(3): 393–9.
85. Michel M, Terriou L, Roudot-Thoraval F, et al. A randomized and double-blind controlled trial evaluating the safety and efficacy of rituximab for warm auto-immune hemolytic anemia in adults (the RAIHA study). Am J Hematol 2017; 92(1):23–7.
86. Reynaud Q, Durieu I, Dutertre M, et al. Efficacy and safety of rituximab in auto-immune hemolytic anemia: A meta-analysis of 21 studies. Autoimmun Rev 2015; 14(4):304–13.
87. Rao A, Kelly M, Musselman M, et al. Safety, efficacy, and immune reconstitution after rituximab therapy in pediatric patients with chronic or refractory hemato-logic autoimmune cytopenias. Pediatr Blood Cancer 2008;50(4):822–5.
88. Maung SW, Leahy M, O'Leary HM, et al. A multi-centre retrospective study of rituximab use in the treatment of relapsed or resistant warm autoimmune hae-molytic anaemia. Br J Haematol 2013;163(1):118–22.
89. Zecca M, Nobili B, Ramenghi U, et al. Rituximab for the treatment of refractory autoimmune hemolytic anemia in children. Blood 2003;101(10):3857–61.
90. Coon WW. Splenectomy in the treatment of hemolytic anemia. Arch Surg 1985; 120(5):625–8.
91. Balague C, Targarona EM, Cerdan G, et al. Long-term outcome after laparo-scopic splenectomy related to hematologic diagnosis. Surg Endosc 2004; 18(8):1283–7.
92. Patel NY, Chilsen AM, Mathiason MA, et al. Outcomes and complications after splenectomy for hematologic disorders. Am J Surg 2012;204(6):1014–9.
93. Hill QA, Stamps R, Massey E, et al. The diagnosis and management of primary autoimmune haemolytic anaemia. Br J Haematol 2017;176(3):395–411.

94. Zupanska B, Sylwestrowicz T, Pawelski S. The results of prolonged treatment of autoimmune haemolytic anaemia. Haematologia (Budap) 1981;14(4):425–33.

95. Worlledge SM, Brain MC, Cooper AC, et al. Immmunosuppressive drugs in the treatment of autoimmune haemolytic anaemia. Proc R Soc Med 1968;61(12): 1312–5.

96. Hershko C, Sonnenblick M, Ashkenazi J. Control of steroid-resistant autoimmune haemolytic anaemia by cyclosporine. Br J Haematol 1990;76(3):436–7.

97. Howard J, Hoffbrand AV, Prentice HG, et al. Mycophenolate mofetil for the treatment of refractory auto-immune haemolytic anaemia and auto-immune thrombocytopenia purpura. Br J Haematol 2002;117(3):712–5.

98. Moyo VM, Smith D, Brodsky I, et al. High-dose cyclophosphamide for refractory autoimmune hemolytic anemia. Blood 2002;100(2):704–6.

99. Pignon JM, Poirson E, Rochant H. Danazol in autoimmune haemolytic anaemia. Br J Haematol 1993;83(2):343–5.

100. Fadlallah J, Michel M, Crickx E, et al. Bortezomib and dexamethasone, an original approach for treating multi-refractory warm autoimmune haemolytic anaemia. Br J Haematol 2019;187(1):124–8.

101. Passweg JR, Rabusin M, Musso M, et al. Haematopoetic stem cell transplantation for refractory autoimmune cytopenia. Br J Haematol 2004;125(6):749–55.

102. Miano M, Calvillo M, Palmisani E, et al. Sirolimus for the treatment of multi-resistant autoimmune haemolytic anaemia in children. Br J Haematol 2014; 167(4):571–4.

103. Markham A. Fostamatinib: First Global Approval. Drugs 2018;78(9):959–63.

104. A Safety and Efficacy Study of R935788 in the Treatment of Warm Antibody Autoimmune Hemolytic Anemia (AIHA) (SOAR). US National Library of Medicine. Available at: https://clinicaltrials.gov/ct2/show/NCT02612558. Accessed November 1, 2021.

105. A Phase 3, Multi-Center, Randomized, Double-Blind, Placebo-Controlled Study of Fostamatinib Disodium in the Treatment of wAIHA. US National Library of Medicine. 2021. Available at: https://clinicaltrials.gov/ct2/show/NCT03764618. Accessed November 1, 2021.

106. Even-Or E, Naser Eddin A, Shadur B, et al. Successful treatment with daratumumab for post-HSCT refractory hemolytic anemia. Pediatr Blood Cancer 2020; 67(1):e28010.

107. Schuetz C, Hoenig M, Moshous D, et al. Daratumumab in life-threatening autoimmune hemolytic anemia following hematopoietic stem cell transplantation. Blood Adv 2018;2(19):2550–3.

108. The Safety of Repurposing Daratumumab for Relapsed or Refractory Autoimmune Antibody Mediated Hemolytic Anemia (DARA-AIHA). US National Library of Medicine. 2021. Available at: https://clinicaltrials.gov/ct2/show/NCT05004259. Accessed November 1, 2021.

109. Manda S, Dunbar N, Marx-Wood CR, et al. Ibrutinib is an effective treatment of autoimmune haemolytic anaemia in chronic lymphocytic leukaemia. Br J Haematol 2015;170(5):734–6.

110. St Bernard R, Hsia CC. Safe utilization of ibrutinib with or without steroids in chronic lymphocytic leukemia patients with autoimmune hemolytic anemia. Ann Hematol 2015;94(12):2077–9.

111. Fang LW, Pan H, Shi J. [Ibrutinib treatment for 2 cases of relapsed/refractory autoimmune hemolytic anemia: a pilot study]. Zhonghua Xue Ye Xue Za Zhi 2020;41(5):412–6.

112. The Safety and Efficacy of Ibrutinib in Refractory/Relapsed Autoimmune Hemolytic Anemia. US National Library of Medicine. 2021. Available at: https://clinicaltrials.gov/ct2/show/NCT04398459. Accessed November 1, 2021.
113. Study to Assess the Safety, Tolerability, Efficacy and PK of APL-2 in Patients With Warm Type Autoimmune Hemolytic Anemia (wAIHA) or Cold Agglutinin Disease (CAD). US National Library of Medicine. Available at: https://clinicaltrials.gov/ct2/show/NCT03226678. Accessed November 1, 2021.
114. A Safety Study of SYNT001 in Participants With Warm Autoimmune Hemolytic Anemia (WAIHA). US National Library of Medicine. Available at: https://clinicaltrials.gov/ct2/show/NCT03075878. Accessed November 1, 2021.
115. ALXN1830 in Patients With Warm Autoimmune Hemolytic Anemia. US National Library of Medicine. Available at: https://clinicaltrials.gov/ct2/show/NCT04256148. Accessed November 1, 2021.
116. Efficacy and Safety of M281 in Adults With Warm Autoimmune Hemolytic Anemia. US National Library of Medicine. Available at: https://clinicaltrials.gov/ct2/show/NCT04119050. Accessed November 1, 2021.

Updates on the Diagnosis and Management of Cold Autoimmune Hemolytic Anemia

Morie A. Gertz, MD, MACP

KEYWORDS

- Cold agglutinin disease • Immune-mediated hemolysis
- IgM monoclonal gammopathy • Waldenström macroglobulinemia

KEY POINTS

- Cold agglutinin disease represents a direct antiglobulin-positive hemolytic anemia.
- In cold agglutinin disease, there is a low-grade lymphoplasmacytic clonal process in the bone marrow that produces a monoclonal IgM protein that fixes complement to the red cell and results in extravascular hemolysis.
- Current therapies focus on the reduction of synthesis of the monoclonal IgM protein using rituximab, bortezomib, or bendamustine alone or in combination.
- Emerging therapy designed to block complement activation such as sutimlimab can result in the resolution of the hemolysis without the use of cytotoxic agents.

INTRODUCTION

Immune-mediated hemolytic anemias can be divided into 2 separate types based on in vitro experiment performed over 80 years ago.[1] The most common form of immune-mediated hemolysis occurs in vitro at 37° so-called warm antibody type hemolytic anemia.[2] This is covered in other chapters in this volume of Hematology Oncology Clinics of North America. The other is cold hemolytic anemia. Patients with this disorder will have agglutination with or without hemolysis at 3 degree centigrade without adding an antiglobulin (Coombs antiserum) to promote the reaction. Patients were previously classified as having primary cold agglutinin disease usually in the context of an IgM monoclonal protein in the serum that serves to fix complement to the red blood cells. A secondary form of cold agglutinin syndrome, generally self-limited and postinfectious, is historically associated with the Epstein Barr virus or with myco-plasma pneumonia and atypical bacterium.[3] In these instances, a polyclonal immuno-globulin M molecule develops as part of the primary immune response to the infection

Mayo Clinic, Two Hundred South West 1st Street, Rochester, MN 55905, USA
E-mail address: gertm@mayo.edu
Twitter: @moriegertz (M.A.G.)

Hematol Oncol Clin N Am 36 (2022) 341–352
https://doi.org/10.1016/j.hoc.2021.11.001
0889-8588/22/© 2021 Elsevier Inc. All rights reserved.

hemonc.theclinics.com

and leads to deposition of complement on the surface of the red blood cell. Some patients will have features of both warm and cold hemolysis with immunoglobulin G and complement on the red cell surface.[4] This category is completed with paroxysmal cold hemoglobinuria whereby an immunoglobulin G molecule capable of activating complement and leading to intravascular hemolysis develops often as a postinfectious phenomenon historically described with syphilis but seen in pregnancy[5] and with viral infections including parvovirus.[6]

Cold agglutinins were identified over 100 years ago long before the concepts of immunoglobulins and complement were developed and before the development of the direct antiglobulin test. The 1st monoclonal antibody ever identified was a cold agglutinin from a patient with cold agglutinin disease. Cold agglutinin antibodies are typically immunoglobulin M but rarely may be immunoglobulin G or rarely immunoglobulin A. The target antigen on the red cell surface to which the immunoglobulin binds is Ii, the so-called individuality blood grouping. In neonates and children, the red cells express i but after the age of 18 months all red cells express I.[7]

PATHOPHYSIOLOGY

Primary cold agglutinin disease is responsible for approximately 15% of all autoimmune hemolytic anemias. Cold agglutinins are auto-antibodies that react optimally at temperatures of 3 to 4 degree centigrade. The patient's serum will agglutinate with all available red cells in a laboratory. The so-called cold agglutinin titer is measured by serial dilutions of the patient's serum by a factor of 2 and the titer is the most dilute serum capable of causing visual agglutination. A clinically significant titer is usually considered greater than 1:64 (2^6 dilution of the patient's serum).[8] Some cold agglutinins will lead to agglutination at higher temperatures. The temperature at which agglutination still occurs is referred to as the thermal amplitude. The higher the thermal amplitude the more clinically significant the agglutinating antibody is.[9] If the thermal amplitude exceeds 28 to 30-degree centigrade red cells will agglutinate in acral parts of the circulation even at mild ambient temperatures and often complement fixation and complement-mediated extravascular hemolysis will ensue.[10]

Because red cells are positively charged, they naturally repel one another and will naturally disperse when viewed on a glass slide. Because immunoglobulin M is a macromolecule with a molecular weight approaching 1 million Daltons, it can bridge the intercellular distance which is seen on a peripheral blood film is agglutination, as distinct from rouleaux formation. The IgM protein is typically glycosylated.[11]

The mechanism underlying hemolysis is well understood. Once IgM binds to the surface of the red blood cell via the I antigen-binding site, complement is fixed to the surface of the red blood cell via the classical complement pathway starting with C1. Theoretically, it would be possible for the alternate complement pathway to activate C3 but in practice, this rarely is seen. In sequence, the activation of complement brings complement components 2, 4, and 3 to the surface of the red cell. At physiologic temperatures, the IgM molecule does not remain on the surface of the red cells. The red cell circulates with the 3rd component of complement on the surface. Naturally occurring C3 convertase removes C3a from the red cell and the cells are now circulating with C3b on the surface. The mononuclear phagocyte system is rich in C3b receptors. This system is found in the spleen, the Kupffer cells of the liver, alveolar macrophages, and lymph nodes. As red cells with C3b on the surface interface with the cells binding C3b removal of small parts of the membrane occurs. As these cells repeatedly pass through, more of the red cell membrane is removed resulting in spherocytes. Ultimately sufficient membrane is removed leading to red cell destruction in the extravascular space. Intravascular hemolysis is generally not seen and when intravascular hemolysis occurs it is associated with a major flare in the intensity of hemolysis often triggered by an infection. The entire circulating red cell mass is not susceptible to hemolysis. Enzymes act on C3b and remove C3c leaving the red cells with a coating of C3d. These cells are resistant to hemolysis as no receptors are found in the mononuclear phagocyte system. Fatal hemolysis is rare because C3d coated red blood cells will not undergo extravascular hemolysis.[12]

CLINICAL FEATURES

In most patients, the hemolysis, when it occurs, is completely extravascular therefore clinical features such as fever, flank pain, and dark urine are lacking as these are typical features of intravascular hemolysis. These patients' clinical features cannot be distinguished from warm immune hemolytic anemia and include indirect hyperbilirubinemia, LDH elevation, reticulocytosis, absent haptoglobin, and spherocytes visible in the peripheral blood film **Fig. 1**.[13] Direct antiglobulin testing is positive and specific IgG and complement antibody testing will be negative for immunoglobulin G and positive for the complement. Artifactual changes may be seen as clumps of red cells pass through the aperture of a Coulter counter-type machine. These would include elevations of the mean corpuscular volume to levels that are not physiologic such as an MCV of more than 130 fL can occur. In addition, wild inaccuracy of the red blood cell count may occur. Artifactually depressed red cell counts as low as 0.5 million per femtoliter can be recorded which results in calculating hematocrits of less than 5%. As the hemoglobin is measured after the red cells are lysed inside the machine the value is quite accurate and may be used for all clinical decision making. The direct

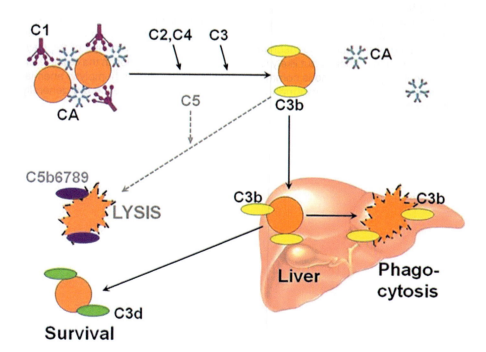

Fig. 1. Pathophysiology of cold agglutinin in disease.

antiglobulin test (Coombs) is positive for complement. In practice, if the Coombs test is negative cold agglutinin hemolysis would be very unusual. Although the hemoglobin will be accurate in a routinely processed specimen, an unwarmed specimen will give spurious results for rbc number, MCV, and hematocrit.[14]

One should expect patients with cold hemagglutinin disease to have a monoclonal IgM protein however, a peak on the serum protein electrophoresis may not occur and the protein may be detectable only by immunofixation reflecting a size less than 0.2 g/dL. The monoclonal protein typically ranges between 0.5 and 1.5 g/deciliter. A bone marrow biopsy should be performed in all patients, and will demonstrate red cell hyperplasia as well as clonal lymphoplasmacytic cells. The number may be sufficient for a pathologist to designate this as lymphoplasmacytic lymphoma but in many cases, the clone is only detectable using immunohistochemical techniques or flow.[15] As in virtually all forms of lymphoplasmacytic lymphoma, if sufficient tumor cells are detected, a mutation in MYD88 will be detected. This is not required for the diagnosis but is confirmatory and supportive. The diagnosis of lymphoplasmacytic lymphoma in the bone marrow and any level of IgM monoclonal protein fulfills the criteria for a diagnosis of Waldenstrom Macroglobulinemia. However, most patients with cold agglutinin disease do not fulfill the consensus criteria for the treatment of macroglobulinemia unless the hemolysis is sufficient to produce symptomatic anemia.[16]

The most common symptomatic manifestation of cold agglutinin hemolytic anemia is symptoms related to the anemia.[17] As in all patients with chronic anemia there is a shift in the oxygen saturation curve due to rising levels of intracellular 2,3 DPG. Therefore, higher levels of oxygen are liberated to the tissues at higher partial pressures of oxygen. In the clinic, one observes well-compensated function and the ability to perform activities of daily living at hemoglobin less than 7 g/deciliter. As red cells circulate through surface veins, they will agglutinate so that flow through the surface vessels is reduced. The deoxygenated agglutinated red cells produce very typical livedo reticularis (**Figs. 2–4**) on the hands and lower extremities that are completely reversible with rewarming of the skin. The mechanism underlying the development of the Raynaud phenomenon is unclear but likely relates to in vivo agglutination in the digits leading to oxygen deprivation and is commonly seen in cold agglutinin hemolytic anemia. Acrocyanosis is a common accompaniment of cold agglutinin disease but generally can be easily managed with cold avoidance.

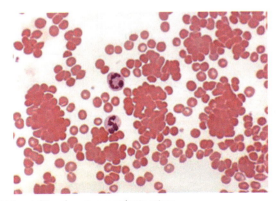

Fig. 2. Peripheral blood film showing agglutination.

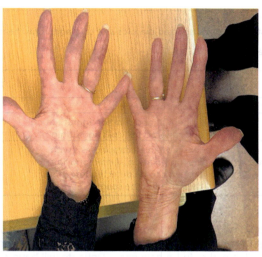

Fig. 3. Livedo reticularis of the hands.

EVALUATION
Laboratory

The list of recommended tests when cold agglutinin hemolytic anemia is in the differential diagnosis can be found in **Table 1**. Specific attention to the mean corpuscular volume for spurious elevation or low hematocrit out of proportion to other parameters is important. The reticulocyte count is typically elevated but, in many instances, whereby the hemolysis is low-grade compensated it may be less than 3%. Due to the loss of membrane from the antibody-coated red cells spherocytes are common. Markers of red cell destruction include elevation of the indirect bilirubin. In all patients that have a positive direct antiglobulin test testing for immunoglobulin G and complement specificity is required. If complement antiglobulin testing is positive cold

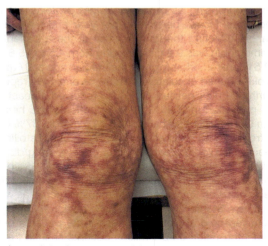

Fig. 4. Livedo reticularis of the lower extremities.

Table 1		
Recommended testing for the suspected diagnosis of cold agglutinin hemolytic anemia		
Tests Recommended for AD Assessment		
CBC	LDH	Quantitative Immunoglobulins
Reticulocyte count	Bilirubin Total and direct	Haptoglobin
DAT	Peripheral Blood film for agglutination and spherocytes; cold agglutinin titer	CH50, C3, C4
-if + IgG & C3 monospecific DAT	serum protein electrophoresis with immunofixation, if no monoclonal protein can be detected infectious causes should be sought	

agglutinin titer should be measured Immunofixation of the serum in urine looking for the monoclonal IgM protein is required. Nonspecific markers of hemolysis including the LDH and haptoglobin should be assessed. Patients will have depression in complement levels and measurement of total hemolytic complement, C3 and C4 are required.

Bone Marrow

When a monoclonal IgM protein is confirmed, a bone marrow examination is indicated. Assessment for the presence of lymphoplasmacytic lymphoma or clonal B cells that do not meet criteria for overt lymphoma is indicated. Genetic studies of the bone marrow include a search for mutation in MYD88 and if a mutation is found, CXCR4 mutation should be sought. If overt lymphoma is found in the bone marrow staging would include imaging for the presence of mediastinal or retroperitoneal lymphadenopathy.

NATURAL HISTORY OF COLD AGGLUTININ DISEASE

A long-term study in Norway identified 232 patients fulfilling criteria for CAD. The median age at onset was 67 years with a range from 30 to 92. The male to female ratio was 0.54 which was surprising as monoclonal IgM proteins are more common in men. The incidence was 1 case per million per year and the prevalence 16 cases per million population-reflecting the long survival of these patients after diagnosis. The mean initial hemoglobin was 9.2 g/dL ranging from 4.5 to 15.6 g. Median survival from onset was 12.5 years remarkably given the median age of 67 at diagnosis. 91% of the patients had cold-induced circulatory symptoms and 74% reported exacerbation of their anemia during febrile illnesses. 51% had received at least 1 red cell transfusion. In an update published in 2020%, 27% of patients had hemoglobin less than 8 g/dL with a mean LDH of 534 and bilirubin of 2.75 mg/dL. 37% of patients had hemoglobin ranging from 8 to 10 g/dL with an LDH of 450 and a bilirubin of 2.5 mg/dL. 36% of patients had hemoglobin greater than or equal to 10 g/dL. In all subsets, the median IgM level was less than 0.7 g per deciliter.[3]

Large studies in the United States are based on artificial intelligence analysis of millions of medical records using keywords in the medical record as well as specific laboratory data.[18] The Stanford translational research integrated database retrospectively identified cold agglutinin disease in 29 patients over 16 years. This database contained information on 2.1 million patients seen in the Stanford system. General observations included disease severity fluctuations that resulted in variable symptoms over time. In some patients, the anemia was mild causing little change in the quality of life. But for some, anemia had a substantial impact on the quality of life with symptoms including acrocyanosis, fatigue, dyspnea, weakness, and mild to severe Raynaud. 79% of patients had severe or moderate anemia. The mean and median hemoglobin levels were 8.3 and 8.2 g/dL and ranged from 4.7 to 11.6 g/dL. 72% of the patients had at least 1 severe anemia event, defined as transfusion required, within the 1st year of monitoring. A subset of patients remained severely anemic despite multiple therapeutic interventions. Overall, there were 7.1 severe anemia events per patient-year, 10.8 moderate events per patient-year, 8.0 mild events per patient-year during the follow-up. 65% of patients had at least 1 transfusion. The median number of transfusions was 4.4 per patient-year of follow-up. The average number of red cell units per transfusion was 1.5.

A previously unsuspected complication was a high incidence of thrombotic events. Of the 29 patients, 5 suffered venous thromboembolism. In 3 there was a portal vein thrombosis and 2 had acute venous embolism of deep vessels.[19]

The largest cohort comes from the Optum integrated claims data set. Using natural language processing and search terms linked to laboratory data, 55,000,000 patients were screened. A total of 608 cold agglutinin disease patients were identified and were matched with 5873 control patients. 70% of patients were more than 65%, 64% were women. 88.8% of patients were Caucasian. Among 255 cold agglutinin disease patients, there were 395 thromboembolic events representing 31.3% of the total cold agglutinin population developing VTE. The control population had an incidence of 20.2%. Among the 31% that developed thrombosis, 18% had 1 event and 13% had more than 1 event. The odds of having a thrombotic event were 1.85 times higher in patients than in controls. The types of venous thromboembolic events were not merely low-risk DVT.[19] Six patients had a portal vein thrombosis, 40 had a pulmonary embolism and 10 had mesenteric thrombosis. There were also 16 arterial emboli in thromboses including 55 myocardial infarctions and 180 for strokes. All of these were statistically more frequent than the controls. I hemoglobin less than 8 g/dL was seen in 23.1%. Hemoglobin from 8.1 to 10 g/dL was seen in 29.5% and 47.4% had hemoglobin greater than 10 g/dL. Abnormal bilirubin or LDH was seen in 91% of patients. Cold agglutinin disease is associated with a significantly increased risk of venous arterial and cerebral thrombotic events. These thrombotic events are not predicted by the severity of the anemia. However, a relationship was noted that patients with thrombotic events had a higher LDH level.

TREATMENT INCLUDING EMERGING THERAPIES FOR COLD AGGLUTININ HEMOLYTIC ANEMIA

The polyclonal postinfectious secondary forms of cold agglutinin hemolysis associated with infectious mononucleosis and mycoplasma pneumonia can be quite severe but are self-limited transient and result in full recovery.[20] Most patients require supportive care only and as this tends to occur in younger individuals with a primary symptom of fatigue, most are misattributed to postinfectious malaise and only the most severe instances with profound anemia come to medical attention with a firm diagnosis. As the primary immune response mediated by immunoglobulin M begins to decline at day 14 full recovery begins.[12]

Unfortunately, monoclonal cold agglutinin disease is associated with the production of an IgM monoclonal protein from lymphoplasmacytic cells in the marrow and results in a chronic sustained relapsing-remitting anemia. Historically, treatment has been directed toward the elimination of the lymphoplasmacytic cells responsible for the synthesis of the IgM protein.[21] Although, in principle, this should result in lesser IgM protein complement fixation on the red cell surface, the reality is attempts to reduce the IgM protein to levels below which hemolysis no longer occurs is quite a challenge. The standard therapies for warm hemolytic anemia including corticosteroids, splenectomy, and intravenous immunoglobulin infusions are typically ineffective: these therapies that tend to affect the interaction between the red cell and the mononuclear phagocyte system, cannot overcome the substantial density of complement on the red blood cells surface There use is, therefore, discouraged in CAD.

Rituximab has been extensively studied in CAD.[22] This agent is well known to produce responses in Waldenstrom Macroglobulinemia; however, it is not very effective in cold agglutinin disease. In the report of 35 patients, 19 (52.3%) has had an initial increase in hemoglobin with a median of 1.5 g/dL. However, and 6 of these 19 had a decline of at least 1.5 g/dL after having an initial response. The rituximab was given 375 mg/M2 for 4 doses LDH and bilirubin was measured in 28 of these patients and in 22 there was a persistent elevation of bilirubin or LDH within 12 months of therapy reflecting that Rituximab as a single agent is not very effective for sustained responses.[23] A recent trial of rituximab reported 13 of 16 patients (81%) responded to the therapy. Responders achieved a median increase in hemoglobin levels of 4.5 g/dL.

Bortezomib also known to be active in the management of lymphoplasmacytic lymphoma was administered to 21 CAD patients with hemoglobin of less than 10 g of whom 10 were transfusion dependent. Nineteen were evaluable for response (1 excluded for pulmonary embolism on day 4). There were only 3 complete responses, 3 partial response for an overall response rate of 32% suggesting therapy for this disease remains inadequate.[24]

Bendamustine plus rituximab is highly active in the management of lymphoplasmacytic lymphoma. A multi-center trial enrolled 45 patients with CAD.[25] Complete responses were seen in 40% partial response in 31% no responses in 29% complete responses had a 76% reduction in the IgM level, partial response had a 74% reduction in the IgM level. It is noteworthy that patients that failed to have any response in hemoglobin still had a 55% reduction in IgM but no impact on hemolysis. The median increase in hemoglobin for complete responders and partial responders was 4.4 and 3.9 g respectively. A reduction in the cold agglutinin titer was only observed incomplete responders. For symptomatic patients and those that are transfusion dependent a trial of rituximab plus bendamustine should be considered a first-line consideration in the management of cold agglutinin hemolytic anemia.

Ibrutinib was reported in 13 patients with cold agglutinin hemolytic anemia 11 of whom fulfilled criteria for lymphoplasmacytic lymphoma and the remainder chronic lymphatic leukemia or small lymphocytic lymphoma. Two patients were MYD 88 mutation positive. Eight of the 10 were previously treated. Seven were transfusion dependent. The median rise in hemoglobin was 5.6 g/L (2.5–10.3) for the 13 patients. There were 12 complete responses and 1 partial response for an overall response rate of 100%. The median time to complete response was 6 months. **Table 2** summarizes some of the reported response rates to therapy for CAD.[26]

COMPLEMENT INHIBITION IN THE MANAGEMENT OF COLD AGGLUTININ HEMOLYTIC ANEMIA

The theory behind the use of complement inhibition in CAD is sound: In CAD the binding of C3b initiates a cascade of events as discussed earlier leading to the clearance of the red cell extravascularly. Upstream inhibition of complement activation would prevent the deposition of C3 on the surface of the red cell. Downstream complement

Table 2	
Response rates reported to therapy for CAD	
Agent	**Response Rate in %**
Rituximab	52–81
Bortezomib	32
Rituximab/Bendamustine	71
Ibrutinib	100
Sutimlimab	87.5

inhibiting agents such as Eculizumab which prevents the activation of C5 has therefore jas a limited I impact on extravascular hemolysis.[27] The antibody TNT 003 in a macrophage cell culture officially blocked C3 deposition on red cells which resulted in the inhibition of phagocytosis in vitro when cold agglutinin plasma was added to suspensions of red cells at concentrations of 100 μg/mL. This in vitro study supported testing of complement inhibition in the prevention of hemolysis.[28]

Sutimlimab is a humanized monoclonal antibody directed against in a phase 3 trial in 24 patients with CAD, whereby three of the 24 patients did not experience a hematologic response. Overall the mean increase in hemoglobin was 2.6 g and a mean level of 11 g/dL was maintained from week 3 to the end of the 26 week study period, transfusion independence was noted in 71% of patients from week 5 to 26, with normalization of mean bilirubin level by week 3.[29] An improvement in quality of life measures was observed, through clinically meaningful reductions in fatigue. Although 92% of patients experienced one adverse event or more, only 38% of these were assessed as being related to Sutimlimab and mostly graded as 1 to 2. It is expected that continuous lifelong therapy would be required in the absence of definitive treatment of the underlying cause.

SPECIAL CONSIDERATIONS-TRANSFUSIONS AND PERI-OPERATIVE MANAGEMENT

Because there is a pan agglutinin, crossmatch of red cells is challenging and can take many hours.[30] It is important to remember that when the anemia is life-threatening it is not necessary to transfuse with crossmatch compatible red cells. If patients have ABO and Rh compatible cells life-threatening anemia leading to cardiovascular decompensation can be prevented. If patients have other Alloantibodies from prior transfusion this will lead to a delayed hemolytic transfusion reaction weeks in the future and the consequences are minimal and the destruction is the transfused red cells only. When patients need transfusions urgently the hematologist in partnership with transfusion medicine may consider transfusing before a crossmatch to preserve the patient's oxygen-carrying capacity.[31]

Surgical procedures carry special risks for patients with cold agglutinin disease. An in-line blood warmer is often used in the operating room to ensure that any transfused red cells are kept at a temperature that would minimize fixation of IgM to the red cell surface.[32] When extracorporeal circulation is required techniques exist for warming of transfused products. In some instances, it is justified to do preoperative plasma exchange to remove as much of the immunoglobulin M from the patient's plasma as possible when surgery is required and there is insufficient time to wait for the effect of chemoimmunotherapy. Preoperative assessment by the hematologist and discussion with the surgeon to clarify the magnitude and duration of hypothermia during the procedure is required for planning. This will determine the need for plasma exchange preoperatively and whether warming equipment for the extracorporeal circuit is required.

PAROXYSMAL COLD HEMOGLOBINURIA

The diagnostic pathway to this extremely rare complement-mediated intravascular hemolytic disorder follows a similar pathway to cold agglutinin disease. These patients will have a positive complement component of the Coombs test. . When complement is found on the red cell surface by positive complement Coombs test, the patient should have a cold agglutinin titer performed. However, if cold agglutination is not seen the patient should be screened for hemoglobinuria, hemosiderinuria, and free hemoglobinemia. In these patients, a Donath–Landsteiner antibody should also be performed. This disorder shares with cold agglutinin disease a direct antiglobulin test positive for complement. However, the antibody specificity rather than being anti-I, is anti-P. The thermal amplitude is usually less than 20° centigrade. Unlike cold agglutinin disease whereby the hemolysis is extravascular due to C3b, in paroxysmal cold hemoglobinuria activation of the C5 through C9 membrane attack complex leading to cell lysis on rewarming (biphasic antibody) is seen. These patients have intravascular hemolysis leading to dark urine, flank pain, fever, and rigors. In a Canadian study, spanning 124 testing years 3 positive tests were seen in adults and 14 in children. Concordance in the interpretation of the testing was poor.[33] These hemolytic episodes can be seen after infection and are often self-limited.{Tiwari, 2020 #106)[34,35]

SUMMARY AND CONCLUSION

Cold agglutinin disease is an extravascular hemolytic process mediated by the presence of a monoclonal IgM protein. The clinical spectrum is quite broad from mild symptomatic compensated hemolysis and manifestations of acrocyanosis to indefinite transfusion dependency. The process is characterized by a complement-specific Coombs positive Hemolytic process. Standard therapies for warm immune hemolytic anemia including corticosteroids, intravenous immunoglobulin infusions, and splenectomy are ineffective. Primary therapy is directed at the suppression of the cells in the bone marrow responsible for the production of the IgM monoclonal protein. Promising studies with the use of complement inhibition as a strategy to interrupt the hemolysis are forthcoming

CLINICS CARE POINTS

- All patients with a positive Coombs test should be screened for complement mediated hemolysis.
- All patients with a positive complement Coombs should be screen for monoclonal IgM protein in the serum with reduced complement level.
- These patients tend to be corticosteroid resistant.
- Specific precautions are required if surgical intervention with general anesthesia is required.

FUNDING

NCI SPORE MM SPORE 5P50 CA186781-04.

CONFLICTS OF INTEREST

Honorarium from Sanofi.
   There are currently no FDA-approved therapies for cold agglutinin hemolytic anemia. All medications mentioned are all off-label.

REFERENCES

1. Das SS, Bhattacharya S, Bhartia S. Clinical and serological characterization of cold agglutinin syndrome in a Tertiary Care Hospital in Eastern India. Asian J Transfus Sci 2015;9(2):173–6.
2. Cermak J, Pisacka M. Autoimmune hemolytic anemia. Vnitr Lek 2018;64(5): 514–9.
3. Berentsen S. New insights in the pathogenesis and therapy of cold agglutinin-mediated autoimmune hemolytic anemia. Front Immunol 2020;11:590.
4. Bass GF, Tuscano ET, Tuscano JM. Diagnosis and classification of autoimmune hemolytic anemia. Autoimmun Rev 2014;13(4–5):560–4.
5. Akpoguma AO, Carlisle TL, Lentz SR. Case report: paroxysmal cold hemoglobin-uria presenting during pregnancy. BMC Hematol 2015;15(1):3.
6. Kuruvilla N, Vinay V, Rajendran R, et al. A rare case of parvovirus B19 infection induced paroxysmal cold hemoglobinuria in an adult female. Cureus 2020; 12(11):e11622.
7. Fattizzo B, Giannotta JA, Serpenti F, et al. Difficult cases of autoimmune hemolytic anemia: a challenge for the internal medicine specialist. J Clin Med 2020;9(12): 3858.
8. Bendix BJ, Tauscher CD, Bryant SC, et al. Defining a reference range for cold agglutinin titers. Transfusion 2014;54(5):1294–7.
9. Barcellini W. New insights in the pathogenesis of autoimmune hemolytic anemia. Transfus Med Hemother 2015;42(5):287–93.
10. Swiecicki PL, Hegerova LT, Gertz MA. Cold agglutinin disease. Blood 2013; 122(7):1114–21.
11. Sidana S, Murray DL, Dasari S, et al. Glycosylation of immunoglobulin light chains is highly prevalent in cold agglutinin disease. Am J Hematol 2020;95(9):E222–5.
12. Gertz MA. How I treat cold agglutinin hemolytic anemia. Clin Adv Hematol Oncol 2019;17(6):338–43.
13. Arthold C, Skrabs C, Mitterbauer-Hohendanner G, et al. Cold antibody autoim-mune hemolytic anemia and lymphoproliferative disorders: a retrospective study of 20 patients including clinical, hematological, and molecular findings. Wien Klin Wochenschr 2014;126(11–12):376–82.
14. Wilen CB, Booth GS, Grossman BJ, et al. Using direct antiglobulin test results to reduce unnecessary cold agglutinin testing. Transfusion 2017;57(6):1480–4.
15. Kosugi S, Watanabe M, Hoshikawa M. Primary bone marrow lymphoma present-ing with cold-type autoimmune hemolytic anemia. Indian J Hematol Blood Trans-fus 2014;30(Suppl 1):271–4.
16. Tanaka H, Hashimoto S, Sugita Y, et al. Occurrence of lymphoplasmacytic lym-phoma 6 years after amelioration of primary cold agglutinin disease by rituximab therapy. Int J Hematol 2012;96(4):501–5.
17. Packman CH. The clinical pictures of autoimmune hemolytic anemia. Transfus Med Hemother 2015;42(5):317–24.
18. Mullins M, Jiang X, Bylsma LC, et al. Cold agglutinin disease burden: a longitu-dinal analysis of anemia, medications, transfusions, and health care utilization. Blood Adv 2017;1(13):839–48.
19. Broome CM, Cunningham JM, Mullins M, et al. Increased risk of thrombotic events in cold agglutinin disease: a 10-year retrospective analysis. Res Pract Thromb Haemost 2020;4(4):628–35.
20. Teijido J, Tillotson K, Liu JM. A rare presentation of epstein-barr virus infection. J Emerg Med 2020;58(2):e71–3.

21. Berentsen S. How I treat cold agglutinin disease. Blood 2021;137(10):1295–303.
22. Murakhovskaya I. Rituximab use in warm and cold autoimmune hemolytic anemia. J Clin Med 2020;9(12):4034.
23. Jia MN, Qiu Y, Wu YY, et al. Rituximab-containing therapy for cold agglutinin disease: a retrospective study of 16 patients. Sci Rep 2020;10(1):12694.
24. Rossi G, Gramegna D, Paoloni F, et al. Short course of bortezomib in anemic patients with relapsed cold agglutinin disease: a phase 2 prospective GIMEMA study. Blood 2018;132(5):547–50.
25. Berentsen S, Randen U, Oksman M, et al. Bendamustine plus rituximab for chronic cold agglutinin disease: results of a Nordic prospective multicenter trial. Blood 2017;130(4):537–41.
26. Barcellini W, Zaninoni A, Giannotta JA, et al. New insights in autoimmune hemolytic anemia: from pathogenesis to therapy stage 1. J Clin Med 2020;9(12):3859.
27. Herbreteau L, Le Calloch R, Arnaud B, et al. Eculizumab, a real-life successful treatment for refractory cold agglutinin-mediated auto-immune hemolytic anemia secondary to lymphoproliferative disorders. Ann Hematol Ann Hematol. 2021 Aug;100(8):2105–6.
28. Shi J, Rose EL, Singh A, et al. TNT003, an inhibitor of the serine protease C1s, prevents complement activation induced by cold agglutinins. Blood 2014; 123(26):4015–22.
29. Roth A, Barcellini W, D'Sa S, et al. Sutimlimab in cold agglutinin disease. N Engl J Med 2021;384(14):1323–34.
30. Das SS, Chakrabarty R, Zaman RU. Immunohematological and clinical characterizations of mixed autoimmune hemolytic anemia. Asian J Transfus Sci 2018;12(2): 99–104.
31. Jager U, Barcellini W, Broome CM, et al. Diagnosis and treatment of autoimmune hemolytic anemia in adults: recommendations from the First International Consensus Meeting. Blood Rev 2020;41:100648.
32. Hasegawa T, Oshima Y, Maruo A, et al. Paediatric cardiac surgery in a patient with cold agglutinins. Interact Cardiovasc Thorac Surg 2012;14(3):333–4.
33. Zeller MP, Arnold DM, Al Habsi K, et al. Paroxysmal cold hemoglobinuria: a difficult diagnosis in adult patients. Transfusion 2017;57(1):137–43.
34. Tiwari AK, Aggarwal G, Mitra S, et al. Applying Donath-Landsteiner test for the diagnosis of paroxysmal cold hemoglobinuria. Asian J Transfus Sci 2020; 14(1):57–9.
35. Lau-Braunhut SA, Stone H, Collins G, et al. Paroxysmal cold hemoglobinuria successfully treated with complement inhibition. Blood Adv 2019;3(22):3575–8.

Complications of Autoimmune Hemolytic Anemia

Surbhi Shah, MBBS, Leslie Padrnos, MD*

KEYWORDS

- COVID-19 • Autoimmune hemolytic anemia • Venous thromboembolism
- Immunosuppressive therapy

KEY POINTS

- In autoimmune hemolytic anemia (AIHA), the presentation and severity of signs and symptoms depend on the acuity of the development of anemia and patients' underlying comorbid conditions.
- Prophylactic utilization of folic acid 1 mg PO daily in patients with hemolytic anemia has been used to prevent deficiency
- The presence of warm autoantibody can interfere with the screening of alloantibodies for blood product selection in the setting of transfusions.
- Cold antibody hemolytic anemia can cause cutaneous ulceration and necrosis
- There are a plethora of infectious complications that could develop following therapeutic interventions and clinicians should have a low threshold for diagnostic work up.

INTRODUCTION

Autoimmune hemolytic anemia (AIHA) is the group of acquired autoimmune conditions resulting from the development of autologous antibodies, typically immunoglobulin G (IgG) or complement proteins, directed against autologous red blood cell antigens resulting in red cell lysis. A range of antibodies can arise, varying by immunoglobulin subtype or specific temperature facilitating interaction between the immune system and red blood cell antigen, leading to the terminology of warm AIHA and cold agglutinin AIHA.

The incidence of AIHA is approximately 1 to 3 per 100,00 people per year[1] with potentially 40% to 50% of cases described as secondary AIHA with an underlying condition including distinct autoimmune disorders, immunodeficiency disorders, lymphoproliferative disorders, or infections.[2] Treatment of AIHA depends on the type of antibody present and the severity of anemia.

Division of Hematology and Medical Oncology, Mayo Clinic Arizona, 5881 E. Mayo Boulevard, Phoenix, AZ 85054, USA
* Corresponding author. 5881 E. Mayo Boulevard, Phoenix, AZ 85054.
E-mail address: Padrnos.leslie@mayo.edu

Hematol Oncol Clin N Am 36 (2022) 353–363
https://doi.org/10.1016/j.hoc.2021.12.003
0889-8588/22/© 2022 Elsevier Inc. All rights reserved.

The correct diagnosis and treatment of AIHA require careful laboratory assessment and clinical monitoring for response. There are a variety of complications that patients can experience associated with AIHA. Prior studies suggest a variety of mechanisms related to hemolysis that may lead to complications including endothelial activation, inflammation, platelet activation, and red blood cell adhesion.[3,4] The complications include symptoms due to the presence of anemia, existence of the antibody impacting blood bank testing, and side effects from specific therapeutic interventions. Additionally, the presence of active hemolysis and its byproducts can lead to organ dysfunction including renal and vascular complications. The likelihood of these different complications can evolve over time from diagnosis through treatment. Clinicians must remain mindful of the potential complications of AIHA, educating patients and families on the possibilities to facilitate open communication throughout treatment.

COMPLICATIONS RELATED TO ACTIVE HEMOLYSIS
Anemia

The symptoms of AIHA at presentation are driven by the degree of anemia. The National Cancer Institute characterizes anemia as mild with hemoglobin 10.0 g/dL to lower limit of normal, moderate with hemoglobin 8.0 to 10.0 g/dL, severe with hemoglobin 6.5 to 7.9 g/dL, and life-threatening when hemoglobin less than 6.5 g/dL.[5] In AIHA that develops slowly over months, the onset of symptoms will be protracted over time. More commonly, AIHA develops rapidly over days to weeks, and in this case, symptom development will be more severe and thus noticeable by the patient and family.

Common symptoms of anemia, and thus AIHA, include fatigue, dyspnea on exertion, or palpitations. Some patients may also demonstrate jaundice, dark colored urine, or splenomegaly.

A study of 60 patients with warm AIHA revealed that 87% presented with at least one symptom of anemia including fatigue or dyspnea. One in 4 patients in this study reported dizziness and 1 in 3 noted signs of hemolysis including jaundice or dark urine. Fifty-two of the patients had undergone imaging at diagnosis with 10% demonstrating lymphadenopathy.[6]

Symptoms can vary depending on the patient's age. A study of 35 children with AIHA revealed a quarter of patients experienced jaundice, fever, or fatigue at diagnosis. Other symptoms included dark urine or conjunctival pallor noted in 14%, and splenomegaly or abdominal pain in 11%.[7] A larger study of 265 children with AIHA reported dark urine in 80% of patients and organomegaly including splenomegaly in 31% or hepatomegaly in 19%. Importantly, 20% of cases included a concomitant diagnosis of infection.[8] As this second study represents children with all types of AIHA the increase in dark urine reflects an increased rate of Donath–Landsteiner hemolytic anemia, or paroxysmal nocturnal hemoglobinuria, hemolytic anemia in children. This type of AIHA typically follows a viral infection.

On the other hand, elderly individuals who develop AIHA may suffer symptoms at a lesser degree of anemia due to its impact on organ function when considering the symptoms of AIHA in the elderly, a study of 10 patients over the age of 75 years with AIHA revealed 70% experienced chest pain, tachycardia, cardiac failure, confusion, or excessive fatigue.[9] The potential for these cardiac or neurologic symptoms reflects the known increased risk of cardiovascular disease as people age.[10]

In summary, treating clinicians need to have a high index of suspicion for the complications related to the presence of anemia or ongoing hemolysis. The symptoms of anemia, or lack of symptoms, at diagnosis can be attributed to the duration and degree of anemia present. Patient age or comorbidities can shape the type and severity of symptoms of anemia at presentation.

Cutaneous Symptoms

Cutaneous complications are rare but possible in AIHA. Cutaneous ulceration and necrosis are seen more often in the setting of cold antibody hemolytic anemia.[11,12] In cold environments, cold antibodies can cause agglutination of red cells in distal extremities. This decreased red cell flow can result in the extremity feeling numb, painful, and cold. This can lead to acrocyanosis, a functional peripheral arterial disease resulting in skin discoloration, and in extreme situations cutaneous necrosis.[13] The demonstration of these symptoms depend on the titer of antibodies present and the temperature range in which they are active, meaning there is a spectrum of if, and how, patients will experience this complication. Cold autoantibodies are able to bind to red blood cells at less than 37° Celsius, typically below 31° Celsius.[14] Management of these symptoms is to avoid cold temperatures and keep extremities, particularly the hands and feet, warm.

Folate Deficiency

Folate, or vitamin B9, is necessary for DNA synthesis and cell proliferation. This vitamin is absorbed in the small bowel and folate deficiency occurs due to inadequate oral intake, malabsorption, medications, or increased situations of increased demand. Deficiency of folate impacts rapidly proliferating cells including hematopoietic cells in the bone marrow, leading to megaloblastic anemia or pancytopenia.[15] Increased folate demand can be seen in pregnancy as well as increased red blood cell turn over.

To address the increased folate demand is seen in pregnancy and breastfeeding, some nations fortified flour with folic acid and recommend supplementation during pregnancy.[16] This is not the only situation whereby prophylactic folate supplementation has been recommended due to increased situational demand.

Increased folate demand is seen in cases of peripheral red cell destruction and abnormal hematopoiesis, such as hemolytic anemia.[17–19] In chronic hemolysis, prophylactic doses of folic acid are recommended at 1 mg oral daily.[20] This supplementation either remedies, or prevents, folic acid deficiency and allows ongoing compensatory erythropoiesis. It is imperative to also be aware of other nutritional deficiencies that can limit erythropoeisis including iron deficiency in the setting of blood loss or B12 deficiency in the setting of malabsorption. While supplementation of these nutrients is not implemented in hemolytic anemia, it is important to remain aware of the possible deficiencies.

In summary, the presence of ongoing hemolysis can place strain on the body with regards to increased folic acid demands due to ongoing erythropoiesis. Supplementation has been recommended in patients with chronic hemolytic anemia, including thalassemia and sickle cell anemia, and is typically recommended during the duration of AIHA to facilitate ongoing erythropoiesis regardless of baseline folic acid level.

Venous Thromboembolism

The association of venous thromboembolism (VTE) in AIHA is well-documented.[21–23] As hemolysis could be seen either in the intravascular or extravascular compartment, the postulated mechanisms for the development of thromboembolism are related to free plasma hemoglobin, depletion of nitric oxide, presence of autoantibodies including antiphospholipid antibodies in some patients, reactive oxygen species, increased proinflammatory cytokines and mediators, endothelial activation as well as the need for splenectomy/postsplenectomy status.

The rates of VTE in patients with AIHA range from 10% to 27%.[1,4,6,23–30] Pulmonary embolism is a more common presentation in this patient population. The rates of VTE are high in patients with autoimmune disorders when they are admitted to the hospital and have been reported to be up to 2-fold higher in patients hospitalized with AIHA.[25,31–33]

Due to the complex pathophysiology involved in the autoimmune hemolytic process, patients suffering from AIHA are at heightened risk for VTE complications. Despite the awareness of increased risk, it is not easy to ascertain which group of patients would benefit from thromboprophylaxis. There is a paucity of literature to support the use of serum biomarkers such as hemoglobin, LDH, leukocyte count, bilirubin, antiphospholipid antibody, and D-dimer as the predictor for VTE.[1,4,23]

Multiple pathophysiological mechanisms have been proposed. These include immune mechanisms such as systemic inflammation leading to cytokine-induced tissue factor expression, endothelial dysfunction and inhibition of Protein C and fibrinolysis systems, NET release and increased levels of VWF, fibrinogen and factor 8., and non -immune mechanisms such as endothelial cell damage leading to the activation of the Virchow's triad by microvesicular shedding, release of plasma free hemoglobin and heme leading to the release of nitric oxide scavenger.[34]

This situation is further complicated by the fact that a proportion of patients might have concurrent autoimmune thrombocytopenia which would make prophylactic anticoagulation a high-risk intervention. Thus, routine anticoagulation prophylaxis is not a standard of care for patients with AIHA unless there are other considerations for thromboprophylaxis such as cancer, hormonal exposure, pregnancy, recent postop status particularly splenectomy, and use of high dose steroids.

In the event of the development of a venous thromboembolic event, the duration of anticoagulation depend on the nature of the event. If the thrombus was provoked by other risk factors as described above, finite anticoagulation should be considered as per the Chest Guidelines.[35] Also, the degree of ongoing hemolysis along with platelet count would guide the decisions, carefully balancing the risks versus benefits of ongoing anticoagulation. There is no data comparing different anticoagulants in the setting and the presence of AIHA does not impact the choice of anticoagulant used.

Although arterial events are less frequently described, complications such as myocardial infarction and stroke are seen in the setting of AIHA particularly with severe anemia.[36,37] The underlying pathophysiological mechanisms are not well understood, perhaps these are precipitated by the degree of anemia leading to poor perfusion hence ischemic complications.

In summary, VTE is one of the more frequent complications of autoimmune hemolytic disease but currently there are no standard guidelines in terms of preventative strategy both in the inpatient as well as outpatient clinical setting. Thromboprophylaxis in the inpatient setting should be considered for patients with AIHA, as in other cases of medically complicated hospitalized patients, whenever the risk of bleeding is low. In the setting of the development of a thromboembolic event, the duration of anticoagulation in patients with ongoing hemolysis is not clear at this point and is at the discretion of the treating provider after 3 months of therapy.

Renal Dysfunction

Ongoing uncontrolled brisk hemolysis over time can lead to acute kidney injury. This can be caused by renal tubular obstruction by hemoglobin cast precipitation, cytotoxicity to proximal tubular epithelium, and intrarenal vasoconstriction due to the depletion of nitric oxide.[38,39]

Several cases of patients with Evans syndrome, a syndrome of AIHA and immune-mediated thrombocytopenia, who developed acute kidney injury with renal biopsy have been reported. Evoked mechanisms included direct cytotoxicity to the proximal tubular epithelium as well as the demonstration of hemosiderin deposition within the renal tubules leading to chronic renal dysfunction[40] due to cast nephropathy. In a pediatric patient with Evans Syndrome and no associated underlying autoimmune condition, the biopsy revealed hemoglobin casts in renal biopsy attributed to intravascular hemolysis.[41] Lastly IgG4-related kidney disease has been recently described. This fibroinflammatory condition whereby IgG4 positive plasma cells infiltrate the tissue with storiform fibrosis, may or may not be associated with elevated IgG4 levels.[42]

Ongoing hemolysis, particularly intravascular hemolysis can, rarely, impact renal function through a variety of mechanisms. Other causes of hemolysis besides autoimmune hemolysis, such as thrombotic microangiopathy (TMA) can more commonly impact renal function. In the setting of hemolytic anemia with renal dysfunction, once TMA is ruled out, AIHA must be considered and a renal biopsy may be necessary to distinguish the cause of renal injury.

COMPLICATIONS RELATED TO HEMOLYTIC ANEMIA MANAGEMENT
Treatment-Associated Complications

While the presence of hemolysis or anemia can cause complications at diagnosis and during treatment, there are also considerations for adverse effects of the treatment itself. As this is an autoimmune process, many of the therapeutics are immunosuppressive. This increases the likelihood, and atypical nature, of infections. Patients on long-term immunosuppressive therapy should be covered with prophylactic antimicrobials to prevent the development of opportunistic infections. In addition to the general increased infectious risk of pharmaceutical complications, each agent carries distinct complication risks including psychosis (steroids), cardiotoxicity (cyclophosphamide), nephrotoxicity (cyclosporine), anaphylaxis (plasma exchange), or neutropenia (mycophenolate). The variety of potential adverse events from therapeutic interventions prompts the need to review common, and uncommon, side effect profiles at initiation and during treatment, especially if the agent is not commonly used in a clinician's practice.

Table 1 provides a summary of the most common side effects associated with therapeutic interventions for AIHA, many of which focus on immunosuppressive therapy.[43] Complications of each therapy are specific to that particular pharmacologic or surgical intervention.

Transfusion Considerations

In the setting of AIHA, occasionally red blood cell transfusions may be necessary for significant anemia while awaiting a response from immunosuppressive therapy. Identifying the ideal red blood cell unit for transfusion can prove difficult in the setting of AIHA due to disruption in the alloantibody screening process by the presence of a warm autoantibody.

The initial test to identify the presence of AIHA is the direct antiglobulin test, detecting the presence of either immunoglobulin or complement bound to the patient's red blood cells. When the DAT is positive, the next step is a process of elution followed by exposure to reagent red blood cells with known antigen expression. In some cases, this elution and reagent red blood cell exposure lead to panagglutination, and only rarely in this situation does an autoantibody react strongly with a specific antigen informing donor red blood cell unit selection.[55] Thus, detecting a clinically significant

Table 1
Common Side Effects associated with Therapeutic Interventions for Autoimmune Hemolytic Anemia

Therapy	Common Side Effects
Steroids[44]	immunosuppression, infection, endocrine abnormalities with hyperglycemia, psychosis and neurotoxicity, myopathy, osteoporosis, aseptic necrosis of bone
Intravenous immunoglobulin[45]	hypersensitivity reaction, increase the risk for thrombosis, hemolysis, asthenia, GI upset with pain and diarrhea, injection site ecchymosis, and pruritus
Rituxan[44,46]	anaphylactic reaction, hematological toxicity, and hypogammaglobulinemia, GI upset, antibody development, increased risk for infections. Rare cases progressive multifocal leukoencephalopathy (PML)
Cyclophosphamide[47]	hematological toxicity, nausea and vomiting, hemorrhagic cystitis, pulmonary toxicity, secondary malignancy, cardiotoxicity
Mycophenolate mofetil[48]	hematological toxicity particularly neutropenia, gastrointestinal toxicity, opportunistic infections, progressive multifocal leukoencephalopathy
Azathioprine[49]	hematological toxicity particularly leukopenia, hepatotoxicity with increased liver enzymes and bilirubin, susceptibility to infections, Sweet syndrome, and PML
Danazol[50]	Asthenia, erythrocytosis, hepatic toxicity, fatigue and depression, interstitial pneumonitis, Steven–Johnson syndrome, increased thrombosis
Cyclosporine[51]	gastrointestinal toxicity, nephrotoxicity
Sirolimus[52]	gastrointestinal toxicity, elevation of liver function tests, hypertriglyceridemia, blood pressure changes, headaches, mucous membrane irritation, hematological toxicity, sinusoidal obstruction syndrome
Plasma exchange[53]	coagulation factor depletion, anaphylactic reactions, transfusion-related acute lung injury, infectious risk, hypokalemia, hypocalcemia, hematin globulin depletion, ACE-inhibitor-related complications (flushing, hypotension, abdominal cramping), vascular catheter complication, citrate induced metabolic alkalosis
Eculizumab[46]	hypertension, peripheral edema, headache and fatigue, skin rash, gastrointestinal upset, hypokalemia, leukopenia, infection with meningococcus, respiratory complication
Splenectomy[54]	encapsulated organism infection such as pneumococcus and meningitis, venous thromboembolism, secondary malignancies, cardiovascular immense and pulmonary hypertension, bleeding at the time of surgery

red blood cell alloantibody proves difficult in the setting of a broadly reactive autoantibody which can mask an antigen-specific alloantibody. Additional laboratory testing is necessary as an alloantibody can be capable of causing hemolytic transfusion reactions if not identified and managed by antigen-negative red cell transfusions.[56] It has been reported that up to 20% to 40% of patients with AIHA may have alloantibodies present in their sera.[57] Additional laboratory testing can be performed to detect alloantibodies in the presence of broadly reactive warm autoantibody is referred to as autoadsorption. In situations when autoadsorption is not effective, alloadsorption technique is performed.[56]

There are reports that concern for masked alloantibodies in the setting of AIHA may be overestimated, leading to detrimental outcomes for patients if necessary red cell transfusions are withheld.[58] In this study of 36 patients with AIHA, 3 were found to have alloantibodies through traditional testing and only one alloantibody required alloadsorption for detection. Therefore, while alloantibody screening may be difficult in the setting of AIHA additional laboratory techniques may be necessary and prove beneficial for comprehensive management of AIHA. Close communication with blood bank colleagues and acknowledgment that additional techniques will require time before resulting is essential.

SPECIAL CONSIDERATIONS
COVID-19

The pandemic has also brought forward a unique presentation and perspective to the patients infected with SARS-CoV-2 (severe acute respiratory syndrome coronavirus 2), particularly those with underlying B cell lymphoid malignancies. There have been several case reports of patients presenting with AIHA either as a presenting symptom or one that developed during the illness.[59–63] Vice versa, there has been some reporting on the outcomes of the patient with AIHA who developed COVID-19 and it does not seem that patients have worse outcomes.[63–68] One study of 7 patients diagnosed with AIHA associated with COVID-19 infection, revealed that 4 of the 7 individuals were found to have an indolent B lymphoid malignancy, indicating an immune dysfunction which may have predisposed the patient to the infection and/or hemolysis.[69] However, in the era of COVID-19 there is published literature suggesting increased severity of disease for patients who have been treated with Rituxan for their underlying rheumatological or hematological conditions.[70,71] The concern is perhaps there is a reduced ability to mount an immunologic response to active COVID-19 infection, or an appropriate immunologic response to the COVID-19 vaccine, following CD-20 lymphocyte modification. Lastly, there have been case reports of the development of AIHA in the setting of COVID-19 mRNA vaccination which was rather responsive to steroids.[72]

CONCLUSION

AIHA is a collection of conditions requiring accurate laboratory diagnosis and careful consideration for management strategies. In addition to the management of anemia, AIHA can be associated with a spectrum of complications that requires the treating clinician to remain vigilant both at presentation and after treatment initiation. These AIHA complications are not only related to the underlying triggering disease or the process of hemolysis but also complications related to medical therapy. Special considerations related to the COVID-19 pandemic include not only the disease associated with the SARS-CoV-2 virus but also the vaccination process and choice of therapy for AIHA.

SUMMARY

AIHA is a group of acquired autoimmune conditions resulting from the development of autologous antibodies directed against autologous red blood cell antigens resulting in red cell lysis. Beyond the presence, severity and duration of hemolysis which can lead to symptomatic anemia, additional complications at presentation and during treatment require a high degree of clinical vigilance. These include cutaneous, thrombotic, renal disorders, and infectious disorders. Complications can be due to the presence of the pathologic antibody itself, the process of hemolysis, or attributed to treatment. Comprehensive management of AIHA requires awareness and assessment of complications at diagnosis, during, and following treatment.

CLINICS CARE POINTS

- The presence of warm autoantibody can interfere with the screening of alloantibodies for blood product selection in the setting of transfusions.
- Working closely with Blood Bank colleagues and appreciating that blood product unit selection may take additional time and testing is essential to facilitate safe transfusions when necessary.
- Cold antibody hemolytic anemia can cause cutaneous ulceration and necrosis.
- Ongoing hemolysis can contribute to renal dysfunction through a variety of mechanisms.
- Venous thromboembolism is a widely recognized complication associated with AIHA but there is no consensus about prophylactic management for this complication.

REFERENCES

1. Barcellini W, et al. Clinical heterogeneity and predictors of outcome in primary autoimmune hemolytic anemia: a GIMEMA study of 308 patients. Blood 2014; 124(19):2930–6.
2. Liebman HA, Weitz IC. Autoimmune Hemolytic Anemia. Med Clin North Am 2017; 101(2):351–9.
3. L'Acqua C, Hod E. New perspectives on the thrombotic complications of haemolysis. Br J Haematol 2015;168(2):175–85.
4. Lecouffe-Desprets M, et al. Venous thromboembolism related to warm autoimmune hemolytic anemia: a case-control study. Autoimmun Rev 2015;14(11): 1023–8.
5. Badireddy M, Baradhi KM. Chronic anemia. Treasure Island (FL: StatPearls; 2021.
6. Roumier M, et al. Characteristics and outcome of warm autoimmune hemolytic anemia in adults: New insights based on a single-center experience with 60 patients. Am J Hematol 2014;89(9):E150–5.
7. Sankaran J, et al. Autoimmune Hemolytic Anemia in Children: Mayo Clinic Experience. J Pediatr Hematol Oncol 2016;38(3):e120–4.
8. Aladjidi N, et al. New insights into childhood autoimmune hemolytic anemia: a French national observational study of 265 children. Haematologica 2011;96(5): 655–63.
9. Zulfiqar AA, Pennaforte JL, Andres E. Autoimmune Hemolytic Anemia in Individuals Aged 75 and Older: A Study of 10 Individuals. J Am Geriatr Soc 2016;64(6): 1372–4.
10. Sniderman AD, Furberg CD. Age as a modifiable risk factor for cardiovascular disease. Lancet 2008;371(9623):1547–9.
11. Lorenzo-Villalba N, et al. Frostbite and Cold Agglutinin Disease: Coexistence of Two Entities Leading to Poor Clinical Outcomes. Medicina (Kaunas) 2021;57(6).
12. Gregory GP, Farrell A, Brown S. Cold agglutinin disease complicated by acrocyanosis and necrosis. Ann Hematol 2017;96(3):509–10.
13. Sinha A, Richardson G, Patel RT. Cold agglutinin related acrocyanosis and paroxysmal haemolysis. Eur J Vasc Endovasc Surg 2005;30(5):563–5.

14. Kenneth Kaushansky ML. Josef Prchal, Marcel Levi, Olivery Press, Linda Burns, Michael Caligiuri, Williams Hematol, in Williams Hematology. New York: McGraw-Hill Education; 2015.
15. Devalia V, et al. Guidelines for the diagnosis and treatment of cobalamin and folate disorders. Br J Haematol 2014;166(4):496–513.
16. De Wals P, et al. Reduction in neural-tube defects after folic acid fortification in Canada. N Engl J Med 2007;357(2):135–42.
17. Liu YK. Folic acid deficiency in sickle cell anaemia. Scand J Haematol 1975; 14(1):71–9.
18. Kennedy TS, et al. Red blood cell folate and serum vitamin B12 status in children with sickle cell disease. J Pediatr Hematol Oncol 2001;23(3):165–9.
19. Reed JD, Redding-Lallinger R, Orringer EP. Nutrition and sickle cell disease. Am J Hematol 1987;24(4):441–55.
20. Baghersalimi A, et al. Assessment of Serum Folic Acid and Homocysteine in Thalassemia Major Patients Before and After Folic Acid Supplement Cessation. J Pediatr Hematol Oncol 2018;40(7):504–7.
21. Ungprasert P, Tanratana P, Srivali N. Autoimmune hemolytic anemia and venous thromboembolism: A systematic review and meta-analysis. Thromb Res 2015; 136(5):1013–7.
22. Solari D, et al. Autoimmune hemolytic anemia and pulmonary embolism: an association to consider. TH Open 2021;5(1):e8–13.
23. Audia S, et al. Venous thromboembolic events during warm autoimmune hemolytic anemia. PLoS One 2018;13(11):e0207218.
24. Pullarkat V, et al. Detection of lupus anticoagulant identifies patients with autoimmune haemolytic anaemia at increased risk for venous thromboembolism. Br J Haematol 2002;118(4):1166–9.
25. Ramagopalan SV, et al. Risk of venous thromboembolism in people admitted to hospital with selected immune-mediated diseases: record-linkage study. BMC Med 2011;9:1.
26. Bongarzoni V, et al. Risk of thromboembolism in patients with idiopathic autoimmune hemolytic disease and antiphospholipid antibodies: results from a prospective, case-control study. Haematologica 2005;90(5):711–3.
27. Baek SW, et al. Clinical features and outcomes of autoimmune hemolytic anemia: a retrospective analysis of 32 cases. Korean J Hematol 2011;46(2):111–7.
28. Hendrick AM. Auto-immune haemolytic anaemia–a high-risk disorder for thromboembolism? Hematology 2003;8(1):53–6.
29. Ho G, et al. Splenectomy and the incidence of venous thromboembolism and sepsis in patients with autoimmune hemolytic anemia. Blood Cells Mol Dis 2020;81:102388.
30. Bylsma LC, et al. Occurrence, thromboembolic risk, and mortality in Danish patients with cold agglutinin disease. Blood Adv 2019;3(20):2980–5.
31. Zoller B, et al. Risk of pulmonary embolism in patients with autoimmune disorders: a nationwide follow-up study from Sweden. Lancet 2012;379(9812):244–9.
32. Yusuf HR, et al. Risk of venous thromboembolism among hospitalizations of adults with selected autoimmune diseases. J Thromb Thrombolysis 2014;38(3): 306–13.
33. Yusuf HR, et al. Risk of venous thromboembolism occurrence among adults with selected autoimmune diseases: a study among a U.S. cohort of commercial insurance enrollees. Thromb Res 2015;135(1):50–7.
34. Capecchi M, et al. Thrombotic Complications in Patients with Immune-Mediated Hemolysis. J Clin Med 2021;10(8).

35. Stevens SM, et al. Antithrombotic therapy for VTE disease: second Update of the CHEST guideline and Expert Panel report. Chest 2021;160(6):e545–608.
36. Kizilirmak F, et al. Evans syndrome with non-ST segment elevation myocardial infarction complicated by hemopericardium. Indian Heart J 2016;68(Suppl 2): S280–3.
37. Jin H, et al. Report of cold agglutinins in a patient with acute ischemic stroke. BMC Neurol 2015;15:222.
38. Lin H, et al. Evans Syndrome with Acute Kidney Injury. Arch Iran Med 2019;22(6): 336–9.
39. Villegas A, et al. Presence of acute and chronic renal failure in patients with paroxysmal nocturnal hemoglobinuria: results of a retrospective analysis from the Spanish PNH Registry. Ann Hematol 2017;96(10):1727–33.
40. Couri FS, Kandula M. A Case of Evans Syndrome with Acute Hemolysis and Hemoglobin Cast Nephropathy. Am J Case Rep 2020;21:e920760.
41. Gonzalez I, et al. Evans Syndrome Complicated by Intratubular Hemoglobin Cast Nephropathy. Case Rep Pediatr 2017;2017:5184587.
42. Gou SJ, et al. Immunoglobulin G4-related Kidney Disease Associated With Autoimmune Hemolytic Anemia. Iran J Kidney Dis 2018;12(4):243–6.
43. Zanella A, Barcellini W. Treatment of autoimmune hemolytic anemias. Haematologica 2014;99(10):1547–54.
44. Birgens H, et al. A phase III randomized trial comparing glucocorticoid monotherapy versus glucocorticoid and rituximab in patients with autoimmune haemolytic anaemia. Br J Haematol 2013;163(3):393–9.
45. Darabi K, Abdel-Wahab O, Dzik WH. Current usage of intravenous immune globulin and the rationale behind it: the Massachusetts General Hospital data and a review of the literature. Transfusion 2006;46(5):741–53.
46. Engel ER, Walter JE. Rituximab and eculizumab when treating nonmalignant hematologic disorders: infection risk, immunization recommendations, and antimicrobial prophylaxis needs. Hematol Am Soc Hematol Educ Program 2020; 2020(1):312–8.
47. Lechner K, Jager U. How I treat autoimmune hemolytic anemias in adults. Blood 2010;116(11):1831–8.
48. Alba P, Karim MY, Hunt BJ. Mycophenolate mofetil as a treatment for autoimmune haemolytic anaemia in patients with systemic lupus erythematosus and antiphospholipid syndrome. Lupus 2003;12(8):633–5.
49. Lawrence Petz GG. Immune hemolytic anemias. 2nd edition. Philadelpha: Churchill Livingstone; 2003.
50. Pignon JM, Poirson E, Rochant H. Danazol in autoimmune haemolytic anaemia. Br J Haematol 1993;83(2):343–5.
51. Emilia G, et al. Long-term salvage treatment by cyclosporin in refractory autoimmune haematological disorders. Br J Haematol 1996;93(2):341–4.
52. Jasinski S, Weinblatt ME, Glasser CL. Sirolimus as an Effective Agent in the Treatment of Immune Thrombocytopenia (ITP) and Evans Syndrome (ES): A Single Institution's Experience. J Pediatr Hematol Oncol 2017;39(6):420–4.
53. Ruivard M, et al. Plasma exchanges do not increase red blood cell transfusion efficiency in severe autoimmune hemolytic anemia: a retrospective case-control study. J Clin Apheresis 2006;21(3):202–6.
54. Kristinsson SY, et al. Long-term risks after splenectomy among 8,149 cancer-free American veterans: a cohort study with up to 27 years follow-up. Haematologica 2014;99(2):392–8.

55. Gehrs BC, Friedberg RC. Autoimmune hemolytic anemia. Am J Hematol 2002; 69(4):258–71.

56. Buetens OW, Ness PM. Red blood cell transfusion in autoimmune hemolytic anemia. Curr Opin Hematol 2003;10(6):429–33.

57. Sokol RJ, et al. Patients with red cell autoantibodies: selection of blood for transfusion. Clin Lab Haematol 1988;10(3):257–64.

58. Yurek S, et al. Precautions surrounding blood transfusion in autoimmune haemolytic anaemias are overestimated. Blood Transfus 2015;13(4):616–21.

59. Capes A, et al. COVID-19 infection associated with autoimmune hemolytic anemia. Ann Hematol 2020;99(7):1679–80.

60. Maslov DV, et al. COVID-19 and Cold Agglutinin Hemolytic Anemia. TH Open 2020;4(3):e175–7.

61. Jacobs J, Eichbaum Q. COVID-19 associated with severe autoimmune hemolytic anemia. Transfusion 2021;61(2):635–40.

62. Jawed M, Hart E, Saeed M. Haemolytic anaemia: a consequence of COVID-19. BMJ Case Rep 2020;13(12).

63. Barcellini W, Giannotta JA, Fattizzo B. Are Patients With Autoimmune Cytopenias at Higher Risk of COVID-19 Pneumonia? The Experience of a Reference Center in Northern Italy and Review of the Literature. Front Immunol 2020;11:609198.

64. Li M, et al. Evans syndrome in a patient with COVID-19. Br J Haematol 2020; 190(2):e59–61.

65. Perez-Lamas L, et al. Hemolytic crisis due to Covid-19 vaccination in a woman with cold agglutinin disease. Am J Hematol 2021;96(8):E288–91.

66. Demir NA, et al. A case of Evans syndrome secondary to COVID-19. Blood Transfus 2021;19(1):85–8.

67. Huscenot T, et al. SARS-CoV-2-associated cold agglutinin disease: a report of two cases. Ann Hematol 2020;99(8):1943–4.

68. Lopez C, et al. Simultaneous onset of COVID-19 and autoimmune haemolytic anaemia. Br J Haematol 2020;190(1):31–2.

69. Lazarian G, et al. Autoimmune haemolytic anaemia associated with COVID-19 infection. Br J Haematol 2020;190(1):29–31.

70. Houot R, et al. Could anti-CD20 therapy jeopardise the efficacy of a SARS-CoV-2 vaccine? Eur J Cancer 2020;136:4–6.

71. Schulze-Koops H, et al. Increased risk for severe COVID-19 in patients with inflammatory rheumatic diseases treated with rituximab. Ann Rheum Dis 2021; 80(5):e67.

72. Brito S, et al. A Case of Autoimmune Hemolytic Anemia Following COVID-19 Messenger Ribonucleic Acid Vaccination. Cureus 2021;13(5):e15035.

Immunotherapy-associated Autoimmune Hemolytic Anemia

Steven R. Hwang, MD[a,b], Antoine N. Saliba, MD[a,b],
Alexandra P. Wolanskyj-Spinner, MD[a,c],*

KEYWORDS

- Immunotherapy • Immune checkpoint inhibitors • Autoimmune hemolytic anemia
- Immune-related adverse event

KEY POINTS

- Immune-related hematologic adverse events increasingly are reported in the literature with expanding use of immune checkpoint inhibitors.
- Diagnosis of immunotherapy-related autoimmune hemolytic anemia (ir-AIHA) requires a high index of clinical suspicion in patients who are treated with immune checkpoint inhibitors.
- Treatment of ir-AIHA can be challenging and may have an impact on the management of the underlying malignancy.

INTRODUCTION

Immunotherapy continues to play an increasingly central role in the management and treatment of cancer. Immunotherapy is a broad term that has included different classes of drugs and therapies, including immune checkpoint inhibitors (ICIs) and chimeric antigen receptor (CAR) T cell therapy. ICIs have revolutionized the therapeutic landscape of oncology and malignant hematology over the past decade, with significant improvement in survival for patients with various malignancies, including metastatic melanoma, lung cancer, renal cell carcinoma, and lymphoma. ICIs have demonstrated a strong antitumor effect through targeting of specific immune checkpoint molecules, such as programmed cell death protein 1 (PD-1), programmed death ligand 1 (PD-L1),

[a] Division of Hematology, Department of Medicine, Mayo Clinic, 200 First street Southwest, Rochester, Minnesota 55905, USA; [b] Division of Medical Oncology, Department of Oncology, Mayo Clinic, 200 First Street Southwest, Rochester, Minnesota 55905, USA; [c] Mayo Clinic Alix School of Medicine, Mayo Clinic College of Medicine and Science, 200 First Street Southwest, Rochester, Minnesota 55905, USA
* Corresponding author. Division of Hematology, Department of Medicine, Mayo Clinic, 200 First Street Southwest, Rochester, Minnesota 55905, USA.
E-mail address: wolanskyj.alexandra@mayo.edu

Hematol Oncol Clin N Am 36 (2022) 365–380
https://doi.org/10.1016/j.hoc.2021.11.002
0889-8588/22/© 2021 Elsevier Inc. All rights reserved.

hemonc.theclinics.com

and cytotoxic T-lymphocyte–associated protein 4 (CTLA-4), leading to up-regulation of innate immune surveillance. As the role of ICIs continues to expand, the number of recognized ICI-associated immune-related adverse events (irAEs) also has increased. The spectrum of involvement of irAEs is broad and can affect almost any organ system due to nonspecific activation of the immune system (**Fig. 1**). More recently, hematologic disorders, including red cell aplasia, cytopenias, acquired hemophilia A, cryoglobulinemia, and autoimmune hemolytic anemia (AIHA), have been recognized in the literature as rare but potentially life-threatening irAEs.[1,2]

Although CAR T cells take advantage of a patient's own T lymphocytes to treat lymphoma, leukemia, multiple myeloma, and other diseases, irAEs typically are not encountered with this modality. Despite the fact that this customized therapy entails the ex vivo transduction of a gene encoding CAR that then directs a patient's T cells against the malignant cells, extensive review of the literature and clinical experience do not reveal a consistent association between CAR T-cell therapy and irAEs, especially AIHA.[3,4] A caveat, however, is that CAR T-cell therapy is a novel therapeutic modality. It remains to be seen if additional reports of autoimmune disease, in general, and AIHAspecifically, will emerge in the future as more and more patients receive this therapy globally. Therefore, the scope of this review is focused on the description of the diagnosis, management, or prognosis of AIHA in the setting of ICI therapy.

The clinical recognition and diagnosis of immune-related hematologic adverse events (ir-h-AEs) can be particularly challenging given the high incidence of cytopenias related to cancer-directed therapies. Early identification of these clinical entities is important, however, because management typically consists of cessation of the offending ICI, with subsequent implications for the underlying malignancy, and initiation of systemic corticosteroid therapy or other immunosuppressant agents. Warm AIHA, in particular, is one of the more commonly reported ir-h-AEs.[1,5] An up-to-date, comprehensive review of the literature on ICI-associated ir-AIHA, including

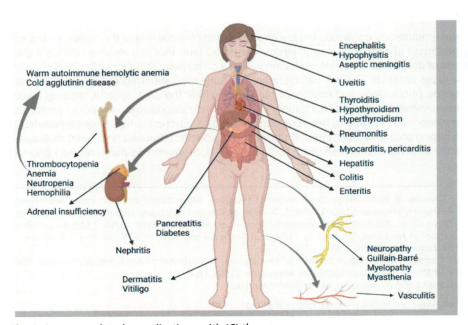

Warm autoimmune hemolytic anemia
Cold agglutinin disease

Thrombocytopenia
Anemia
Neutropenia
Hemophilia

Adrenal insufficiency

Pancreatitis
Diabetes

Nephritis

Dermatitis
Vitiligo

Encephalitis
Hypophysitis
Aseptic meningitis

Uveitis

Thyroiditis
Hypothyroidism
Hyperthyroidism

Pneumonitis

Myocarditis, pericarditis

Hepatitis

Colitis

Enteritis

Neuropathy
Guillain-Barré
Myelopathy
Myasthenia

Vasculitis

Fig. 1. Immune-related complications with ICI therapy.

epidemiology, pathophysiology, classification, clinical diagnosis, management, long-term outcomes, and risk of recurrence upon ICI rechallenge, is presented.

DESCRIPTION OF IR-AIHA EPIDEMIOLOGY
Epidemiology

AIHA is a rare disorder, with a prevalence of approximately 17 cases per 100,000 individuals.[6–9] The exact frequency of AIHA with ICI therapy is difficult to ascertain because of underdiagnosis, clinical heterogeneity, and increasing prevalence with the expansion of ICI use. Underdiagnosis likely is related to several factors.[2,10–26] For instance, in many patients receiving ICI therapy for cancer, anemia may be attributed to other concomitant risk factors like concurrent chemotherapy or radiation therapy use, nutritional deficiency in the setting of cancer cachexia, inflammation, clonal antibody production with lymphoproliferative disorders, and metastatic disease. In addition, given the rise of ICIs as effective anticancer therapies in the past decade, these medications are relatively novel. Particularly in the early days of immunotherapy in clinical practice, many oncologists and medical providers were not familiar with the whole gamut of immune-related complications associated with ICIs. A prerequisite for considering an item on the differential diagnosis list is awareness of that specific complication and its risk factors. Laboratory factors leading to underdiagnosis include the fact that 5% to 10% of patients with clear clinical evidence of AIHA have a negative direct antiglobulin test (DAT), despite using different methods, including the tube method, the more sensitive gel method, the microcolumn method, and washes with cold or low-ionic saline solutions.[27,28] Both improved recognition of AIHA as a complication of ICIs and expansion of their indications in various malignancies have driven an increase in its prevalence. Based on a review of the US Food and Drug Administration (FDA) database as reported in 2019, AIHA in the setting of ICI therapy represented 0.06% to 0.25% of all adverse events reported, occurring more commonly with PD-1 or PD-L1 targeting agents than with CTLA-4 inhibitors.[2] The underlying cancer types mainly were melanoma (41%), non–small cell lung cancer (26%), renal cell carcinoma, Hodgkin lymphoma, and skin cancers.[2] Most cases were IgG-positive warm AIHA, and cold agglutinin disease (CAD) was diagnosed less frequently.[2]

Based on the authors' review of the literature, various ICI agents have been associated with AIHA. The agents reported most commonly associated with AIHA include pembrolizumab, nivolumab monotherapy, ipilimumab and nivolumab combination therapy, ipilimumab monotherapy, and atezolizumab.[1,2,5,20,29] Because the literature search included mostly case series and case reports, it is difficult to ascertain the true prevalence or relative risk of AIHA with the use of different ICI agents. **Table 1** summarizes the larger case series of AIHA with ICI therapy reported in the literature. Although most diagnoses of AIHA were made within 100 days of initiation of therapy with ICIs, cases were reported as early as after 1 cycle and as late as after 39 cycles of therapy.[1,2]

Etiology and Classification

The pathophysiologic premise for ICI–associated ir-AIHA most likely is related to increased immune surveillance. This mechanism of action should be distinguished from other drug-induced AIHAs, where 2 pathophysiologic processes may contribute to hemolysis: (1) binding of autoantibodies to red blood cells (RBCs) only in the presence of the drug through a hapten mechanism and (2) complement-mediated destruction in the presence of the drug through a ternary complex mechanism.[30] Warm AIHA is characterized by antibody-dependent cytotoxicity, mediated by cytotoxic CD8$^+$ T cells and natural killer cells, because the main site of destruction is of RBCs is the

Table 1
Summary of published case series of immune-related auto-immune hemolytic anemia

Case Series (Source)	Number of Patients (n)	Malignancies (n or %)	ICI Used (n or %)	Median Number of Cycles (Range)	Disposition of ICI (% of n)	Treatment of ir-AIHA (n or %)	Outcome of ir-AIHA (n or %)	Disposition of ICI after ir-AIHA resolved (n or %)	ICI Continued Outcomes (n or %)	ICI Rechallenged Outcomes (n or %)
Tanios et al, 2018 (FDA database)	68	Melanoma (32) NSCLC (24) HL (2) RCC (2) Breast (2) Ovarian (1) Not reported/other (5)	Nivolumab (31) Pembrolizumab (13) Ipilimumab/Nivolumab (12) Ipilimumab (7) Atezolizumab (5)	NA	NA	NA	NA	NA	NA	NA
Tanios et al, 2018 (Literature review)	12	NSCLC (6) Melanoma (4) HL (1) Urothelial (1)	Nivolumab (8) Pembrolizumab (2) Ipilimumab/Nivolumab (2)	5.5 (1-39)	NA	Steroids (8) Steroids plus rituximab (2) Steroids plus IVIG (2) Rituximab (1)	CR (9) PR (1) NR (2)	NA	NA	NA
Delanoy et al, 2019 (French pharmaco-vigilance databases)	9	Melanoma (4) NSCLC (3) RCC (2)	Nivolumab (8) Pembrolizumab (1)	2 (1-21)	Held (100%)	Steroids (4) Steroids plus rituximab (5)	CR (6) NR (3)	Rechallenged (1) Discontinued (8)	NA	No recurrent irAE (1)
Leaf et al, 2019 (Multi-center case series)	14	Melanoma (9) NSCLC (3) Colorectal (1) AML (1)	Pembrolizumab (6) Ipilimumab/Nivolumab (4) Nivolumab (3) Ipilimumab (1)	3.5 (1-12)	Held (79%)	Steroids (12) Steroids plus rituximab (1) Steroids plus IVIG (1)	CR (12) PR (2)	Continued (3) Rechallenged (4) Discontinued (7)	CR, Recurrent ir-AIHA (1) PR, recurrent ir-AIHA (1) CR, recurrent non-heme irAE (1)	No recurrent irAE (4)

Study	Cancer type	Agent	Cycles	ICI	Treatment	Response	ICI disposition	Outcome	Recurrence
Kramer et al, 2021 (Multi-center case series)	8	Not reported	Nivolumab (3) Ipilimumab/ Nivolumab (2) Pembrolizumab (1) Ipilimumab (1) Pembrolizumab/ Ipilimumab (1)	2 (1-10)	Held (78%)	Steroids (4) Steroids plus IVIG (1) Steroids plus IVIG and rituximab (1) Steroids plus alemtuzumab (1) Not reported (1)	CR (5) PR (3)	Continued (1) Rechallenged (2) Discontinued (5)	PR, no recurrent irAE (1)	Recurrent ir-AIHA (1) Recurrent non-heme irAE (1)
Saliba et al, 2021 (Single-center case series)	7	NSCLC (3) Melanoma (2) Pancreatic (1) Esophageal (1)	Pembrolizumab (7)	5 (3-15)	Held (86%)	Steroids (6) Steroids plus IVIG (1)	CR (5) PR (3) NR (2)	Continued (1) Rechallenged (3) Discontinued (3)	CR, no recurrent irAE (1)	Recurrent ir-AIHA (3)
Aggregate of all Case Series	118	Melanoma (49%) NSCLC (37%) HL/AML (4%) GU (4%) GI (3%) Breast (2%) Ovarian (1%)	Nivolumab (45%) Pembrolizumab (25%) Ipilimumab/ Nivolumab (17%) Ipilimumab (8%) Atezolizumab (4%) Other (1%)	3 (1-39)[a]	Held (87%)	Steroids (69%) Steroids plus rituximab (16%) Steroids plus IVIG (10%) Other (6%)	CR (68%) PR (18%) NR (7%)	Continued (13%) Rechallenged (26%) Discontinued (61%)	Recurrent irAE (60%) No recurrent irAE (40%)	Recurrent irAE (50%) No recurrent irAE (50%)

[a] Available in 44 patients

spleen and the lymphoid organs.[31] Other pathophysiologic mechanisms involve imbalance of CD4+ regulatory T cells and autoreactive cellular effectors, including activated macrophages via Fc receptor phagocytosis of RBCs opsonized by autoantibodies and complement and T cells.[8]

AIHA can be encountered in association with B-cell malignancies, autoimmune diseases, or drugs.[32] Although drug-induced AIHA is uncommon, the list of drugs that may cause it is expanding.[33] Drug-related antibodies may be drug-independent or drug-dependent. Drug-independent antibodies can be detected in vitro in the absence of the implicated drug. Drugs commonly associated with AIHA mediated by drug-independent antibodies include methyldopa and fludarabine. Drug-dependent antibodies are directed against epitopes on (1) the drug or its metabolites, known as a hapten reaction, or (2) a combination of the drug and the RBC membrane. The drug binds to the RBC surface and becomes part of the antigen. Therefore, drug-dependent antibodies only react in vitro in the presence of the drug. Hapten reactions can be subdivided further into several types. The penicillin type involves a drug that remains on the RBC membrane as a prerequisite for antibody binding. Cephalosporins and penicillin typically cause hemolysis via this mechanism. The immune complex type involves the formation of immune complexes that bind the RBCs then cause complement activation. The passive adsorption type is associated with the administration of antibody preparations like intravenous immune globulin (IVIG). The preparations contain immune complex–type alloantibodies that can react with the recipient's RBC antigens causing alloimmune hemolysis.

Although the precise pathophysiology of AIHA associated with ICI therapy has not been studied extensively and remains unclear, it is believed that the process is related to immunologic dysregulation. When engaged by antibody cross-linking or binding to B7, CTLA-4 dampens the immune response mainly by inhibiting T-cell activation (1) regardless of apoptotic signals and (2) through the restriction of T-cell transition from the G1 phase to the S phase in the cell cycle.[34] PD-1 and its ligands PD-L1 and programmed death ligand 2 (PD-L2) maintain peripheral immune tolerance.[35] They mediate quiescence of mature autoreactive T cells that have escaped central tolerance in the thymus.[35] A tumor overexpressing the function of PD-L1 protects itself from cell killing mediated by CD8+ cytotoxic T cells.[36,37] To counteract this immune tolerance, B7-1, a protein expressed on activated T cells and other antigen-presenting cells, causes down-regulation of the effector T-cell activation by interacting with the PD-L1 on tumor cells.[37] Inhibiting these endogenous immune checkpoints unleashes the immune response against tumors and occasionally against normal cells. Whether autoreactive T cells or autoreactive antibodies are the main driver of many irAEs remains unknown and may not be consistent across different complications. AIHA with ICI is unlikely to be mediated by adsorption to RBC membrane and development of autoantibodies. It also is unlikely that there is cross-reactivity between the drug neoantigen and a red cell antigen. The more likely explanation revolves around immune system activation with subsequent autoantibody formation, blunting of the activity of regulatory T cells, and awakening of quiescent T-cell clones (**Fig. 2**). In a recent publication, among the 127 patients who had either DAT or alloantibody testing prior to ICI initiation, there was no association between DAT positivity before ICI and development of irAEs.[38] Further research is needed to elucidate the pathophysiologic mechanisms underpinning the development of ir-AIHA.

AIHA can be (1) primary, when no association with a secondary cause can be established, or (2) secondary, when an underlying disorder is suspected to be driving the hemolytic process. Secondary causes include lymphoproliferative disorders, autoimmune disease, medications (including antimicrobial agents, such as piperacillin, and

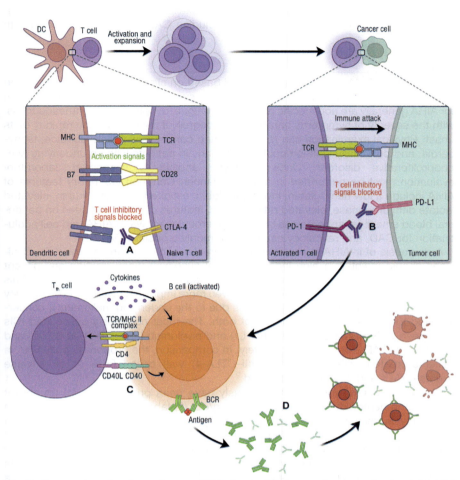

Fig. 2. Proposed mechanisms of warm AIHA due to ICI therapy. Immune checkpoint inhibitors inhibit T-cell–negative costimulation to unleash antitumor T-cell responses directed against tumor antigens. CTLA-4 inhibitors, such as ipilimumab, are anti–CTLA-4 antibodies that block the interaction between CTLA4 and B7, facilitating the activation of T cells (*A*). The interaction between PD-1, expressed on activated T cells, and PD-L1, expressed on tumor cells, dampens the function of T cells. PD-1 inhibitors, such as pembrolizumab and nivolumab, and PD-L1 inhibitors, such as atezolizumab, block the interaction between PD-1 and PD-L1, facilitating the activation of T cells (*B*). T-cell–mediated regulation of the humoral immune system is believed to have an important role in loss of self-tolerance in ir-AIHA. Activated helper T cells stimulate B cells (*C*) to secrete autoantibodies directed against RBCs (*D*). The interaction between the RBC antigen-binding B cell with a helper T cell leads to the expression of CD40L on the helper T cell (T$_{fh}$), and secretion of interleukins stimulate further proliferation of B cells and differentiation into auto-antibody–secreting plasma cells. Blue antibodies denote pharmacologic monoclonal antibodies acting as ICIs. Green antibodies denote autoantibodies produced by activate B cells. BCR, B-cell receptor; DC, dendritic cell; MHC, major histocompatibility complex; TCR, T-cell receptor.

chemotherapy agents, such as fludarabine and oxaliplatin), infection, or other malignancies.[39-41] Warm AIHA and cold AIHA, including CAD, have been reported with ICI therapy.[1,17]

Diagnosis

A diagnosis of AIHA generally is suspected based on clinical findings and confirmed with laboratory evaluation.[42] Common clinical symptoms warranting investigation for AIHA generally are nonspecific and include fatigue, dyspnea, and lightheadedness, with the severity of symptoms paralleling the degree of anemia and the rapidity of its onset. Physical examination can reveal skin and conjunctival pallor, jaundice, tachycardia, and potentially splenomegaly, particularly in patients with an underlying lymphoproliferative disorder. Once hemolytic anemia is suspected, laboratory evaluation must be performed in a timely manner. Common laboratory features of AIHA include a low hemoglobin, low haptoglobin, elevated indirect bilirubin, elevated lactate dehydrogenase, elevated reticulocytes, features of hemolysis seen on peripheral blood smear (ie, spherocytes or microspherocytes for warm AIHA, red cell agglutination for CAD, and reticulocytes), and commonly a positive DAT.

A diagnosis of ir-AIHA is seen within the greater context of the many irAEs. Clinicians should maintain a high index of clinical suspicion when treating any patient with an ICI and a low threshold for initiating diagnostic evaluation for irAEs.[42] This also applies to other ir-h-AEs, and may be even more important given the commonality of cytopenias in patients treated with ICIs due to the underlying malignancy, cancer-directed therapies, or a combination of both. The most commonly associated ICIs were seen with atezolizumab (anti–PD-L1) and nivolumab (anti–PD-1), at 0.25% and 0.21% of all irAEs reported, respectively. In comparison, the proportion of ir-AIHA in patients treated with ipilimumab (anti–CTLA-4) was only 0.06% of all adverse events—irAEs and otherwise—reported.[2]

Diagnostic criteria for ir-AIHA previously have been proposed as (1) an abrupt decrease in hemoglobin by greater than 2 g/dL; (2) laboratory features suggestive of hemolysis, including elevated lactate dehydrogenase and low haptoglobin; (3) temporal association of AIHA after initiation of ICI; (4) exclusion of other causes of acute anemia; and (5) ICI therapy, considered the most likely etiology of AIHA.[20] There appears to be a relatively high prevalence of DAT-negative AIHA in patients diagnosed with ir-AIHA compared with nonICI-associated ir-AIHA, reported as high as 27% to 38% in 1 aggregate cohort review of 31 cases.[20] The proposed reason for this discrepancy could be antibody-independent mechanisms RBC destruction, such as ICI-induced proinflammatory states leading to direct macrophage phagocytosis of RBCs, in a fashion similar to hemophagocytic lymphohistiocytosis. Further studies are needed, however, to investigate for any differences in pathophysiology of DAT-positive and DAT-negative ir-AIHA. None of the patients identified in that particular study underwent enhanced DAT testing, so the true prevalence of DAT-negative ir-AIHA may be lower and closer to the prevalence of that seen in general AIHA.[20]

In CAD, the primary clinical symptom, in addition to those discussed previously related to hemolysis, is cold-induced acrocyanosis, Raynaud phenomenon, or livedo reticularis.[43] Initial evaluation for CAD is similar to that detailed previously for warm AIHA. DAT is positive, however, for the complement component C3b and generally negative for immunoglobulin. Diagnostic criteria for ir-CAD are even more difficult to delineate than those for warm ir-AIHA, primarily due to the paucity of reported cases. Given this, the authors recommend using similar diagnostic criteria to those for non–ICI-associated CAD, with the important additional history of exposure to an ICI as a required criterion.

Treatment

Management of warm AIHA is centered around decreasing the production of IgG autoantibodies with early use of prednisone as first-line therapy.[44] The administration route is dependent on the severity of presentation, with intravenous methylprednisolone reserved for acute presentations with or without hemodynamic instability or inability to tolerate medications enterally; otherwise, oral prednisone, 0.5 mg/kg to 2 mg/kg with a prolonged taper, can be used.[42,45,46] The initial response rate is reported as approximately 70% to 80%,[45] with up to 20% to 40% of patients achieving a durable remission.[47] The remainder subsequently have a chronic, relapsing course requiring subsequent lines of therapy.[45,48] In particularly severe initial presentations of warm AIHA, IVIG also can be used as adjunctive therapy.[49]

Historically, splenectomy has been considered second-line therapy for cases that did not respond to steroids[50] but is associated with poor long-term cure rates of only approximately 20% and increased risks of complications, including infections secondary to encapsulated bacteria in up to 3.3% to 5.0% of patients.[51,52] Rituximab has emerged more recently as the preferred agent for second-line treatment in these patients.[32,53,54] In relapsed/refractory warm AIHA previously treated with steroids, the overall response rate with rituximab is approximately 70% to 80%, with a median duration of response of 1 year to 2 years.[55,56] Most patients respond within 4 weeks after initiation of rituximab.[55,56] Rituximab also has been investigated as first-line therapy in warm AIHA in prospective randomized phase III trials as combination therapy with steroids.[57,58] Both these aforementioned studies showed that addition of rituximab to steroid therapy resulted in nearly identical outcomes with a significantly higher overall response rate (75% vs 31%–36%,), complete response (34% vs 16%), and longer duration of response.[57,58] Given these rates, some hematologists consider using rituximab in the first-line setting for management of warm AIHA. Given its significant side-effect profile, however, notably risk of infection with hypogammaglobulinemia; neutropenia; and risk of reactivation of underlying infections, such as hepatitis B, HIV, and tuberculosis, rituximab—particularly in an often already immunocompromised group of patients—still the is most used in the second-line setting.[46] The most common dose of rituximab used in standard practice is 375 mg/m^2 per week for 4 weeks. Other doses, including 1 g every 2 weeks for 2 doses and 100 mg per week for 4 weeks, have been used with relatively similar response rates, although direct comparisons have not been made.[46]

In particularly severe or refractory cases of warm AIHA, other immunosuppressive therapies have been studied, such as azathioprine, cyclophosphamide, mycophenolate mofetil, and cyclosporine.[59–62] Data assessing overall response rate have been limited, however, to retrospective studies, case series, and case reports. Overall response to those agents, with the caveat of selection for a more refractory subset of warm AIHA, is relatively poor, with a reported overall response rate of approximately 30% to 50%.[59–62] Novel therapeutic agents, such as fostamatinib (spleen tyrosine kinase inhibitor), daratumumab (anti-CD38 antibody), ibrutinib (Bruton tyrosine kinase inhibitor), and alemtuzumab (anti-CD52 antibody), are actively being investigated for potential roles in refractory cases of warm AIHA, with several randomized clinical trials ongoing at this time.[27,63,64]

The treatment of CAD differs greatly from that of warm AIHA. This distinction underscores the importance of establishing a correct clinical diagnosis prior to initiation of first-line therapies. Current therapies for CAD rely on the 2 major bedrocks of the pathogenesis: (1) clonal B-cell lymphoproliferation and (2) complement-mediated hemolysis. The role of steroids is limited in CAD, with a reported remission rate of less than

20% and requirement for high maintenance doses to sustain remission in the few patients who respond.[43,46,65] The role of splenectomy also is limited due to the predominant location of extravascular hemolysis in CAD being the liver.[66,67] B-cell–directed therapies, such as rituximab, have shown promise in several observation studies and a few prospective, nonrandomized trials.[43,68] Given this, rituximab is well-established as first-line therapy in CAD, with a standard dose of 375 mg/m^2 per week for 4 weeks.[54,63] In addition, in the setting of recurrence, retreatment often succeeds in achieving a second response.[69] A prospective trial investigated the addition of bendamustine to rituximab as first-line treatment of CAD and showed an overall response rate of 71%, with a prolonged median response duration of greater than 88 months, sustained for longer than 5 years in 77% of responders, although there was a moderate incidence of grade 3 to grade 4 toxicities noted.[43,70] Given these results, it is reasonable to add bendamustine to patients who do not show response to rituximab early in the treatment course.

The management of ir-AIHA has not been well established, mostly due to the overall rarity of this clinical entity. Therefore, treatment is based primarily on expert guidelines, case series, and reviews of the literature.[42] Glucocorticoids, such as intravenous methylprednisolone and oral prednisone (depending on the severity of the initial presentation), appear to be reasonable first-line options due to the presumed pathophysiology of warm ir-AIHA, as described previously, with the goals of decreasing production of IgG autoantibodies and slowing the rate of RBC destruction. In addition, cessation of the ICI generally is recommended in the setting of active warm ir-AIHA. In patients who do not respond to initial treatment with glucocorticoids, use of rituximab at a similar dose used for treatment of non–ICI-associated warm AIHA is the recommended second-line therapy. Review of the reported cases available in the literature shows an overall response rate of approximately 57% to 75% of patients treated with steroids with or without rituximab.[43,70] In cases of warm ir-AIHA refractory to steroids and rituximab, other immunosuppressive agents used in warm AIHA can be considered, although there are no studies to suggest a preferred agent and clinicians would need to decide on a case-by-case basis. Treatment of ICI-associated immune-related CAD (ir-CAD) is even less well defined, given the paucity of published cases. The authors' recommendation is to use a treatment algorithm similar to that of non–ICI-associated CAD, described previously for ir-CAD. Additionally, for CAD associated with ICI, caution must be exercised to avoid adding an alkylating agent, such as bendamustine, if other chemotherapy drugs are administered concomitantly—especially in patients with cytopenias related to the myelosuppressive effects of cytotoxic therapy. For patients with responding or stable cancer while CAD is progressing, a short interruption or pause in other chemotherapeutic agents is reasonable while the hemolysis is addressed. A proposed algorithm for the management of ir-AIHA is presented in **Fig. 3**.

Prognosis

The overall initial response rate of patients with ir-AIHA is reported to be approximately 57% to 75% with use of first-line and second-line agents, including steroids and rituximab, acknowledging the limited number of cases and lack of substantial follow-up.[2,5,20] Rechallenging with an ICI in patients with previous but resolved irAE has been discussed in prior studies, with review of the recent literature suggesting retrialing ICIs as long as patients are monitored closely.[71] In cases of ir-AIHA, in particular, Hwang and colleagues[15] reported a case of a patient who developed ir-AIHA in the setting of metastatic melanoma treated with ICI and who subsequently was rechallenged with ICI therapy on 2 separate occasions and developed recurrence of ir-

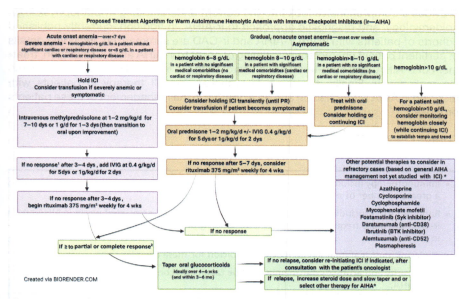

Fig. 3. Proposed treatment algorithm for AIHA with ICIs. (1) Response defined as an increase in hemoglobin of 1 g/dL or greater without dependence of blood transfusions. (2) Achieving partial response (PR) defined as a hemoglobin greater than 10 g/dL but less than 12 g/dL and 2 g/dL above the nadir without blood transfusion. (3) Complete response defined as a hemoglobin of greater than or equal to 12 g/dL and 2 g/dL above the nadir without blood transfusion. BTK, Bruton tyrosine kinase. Created with BioRender.com.

AIHA both times. Leaf and colleagues[20] reported, however, that of the 14 patients in their study, 4 (29%) were rechallenged with ICI, with none having recurrence of AIHA, and 3 (21%) were continued on ICI throughout initial ir-AIHA diagnosis, all 3 of whom had subsequent recurrence of ir-AIHA or other irAE (hepatitis, acute kidney injury, or ICI-associated immune-related *immune* thrombocytopenic purpura.[20] In a literature review by Delanoy and colleagues,[5] only 1 of the 9 patients with ir-AIHA reported underwent rechallenge with ICI, and that patient did not experience recurrence of AIHA. Overall, it appears that rechallenge with ICI in patients with resolved ir-AIHA can be trialed, particularly if alternative cancer-directed therapies are suboptimal to treatment with ICI, with strong recommendations for close and frequent monitoring of clinical and laboratory parameters. In addition, alternative etiologies of both hemolytic and nonhemolytic anemia must be considered when monitoring for recurrence, particularly if there are concurrently administered cytotoxic medications, evidence of metastatic bone marrow involvement, or secondary malignancies involving the bone marrow, such as therapy-related myeloid neoplasms.

SUMMARY

Immunotherapy has changed the therapeutic landscape of malignant hematology and oncology. As immunotherapy—ICIs, in particular—become used more widely, the number of reported irAEs also is increasing. A growing number of ir-h-AEs, including warm ir-AIHA and ir-CAD, are recognized as clinically important entities with challenging diagnostic and management decisions in practice. This review provides a comprehensive look into the current understanding of pathophysiology, epidemiology, and diagnostic approach to ir-AIHA. In addition, currently published cohorts of patients with warm ir-AIHA and ir-CAD are summarized, including details of pertinent patient characteristics, timing of onset to ir-AIHA after ICI initiation, treatment of ir-AIHA, and long-term outcomes of both the irAE and the patient's underlying malignancy. Finally, the topic of rechallenging ICI therapy in patients with resolved ir-AIHA is touched on and an algorithm in the management of these patients proposed.

CLINICS CARE POINTS

- Immunotherapy including the use of ICIs are becoming more popular in the management of a greater number of malignancies.
- Reported irAEs including Hematologic complications such ICI-associated warm ir-AIHA and ir-CAD, are more frequent, and present challenging diagnostic and management decisions in practice.
- Clinicians must maintain a high index of suspicion for these complications.
- The severity and acuity of the anemia must be taken into consideration in the management of ir-AIHA.
- Standard front-line therapy for ir-AIHA includes the use of steroids upfront, as well as consideration of the addition of Rituximab or IVIG. There is no consensus in the management of refractory or relapsed disease.
- Decisions regarding the disposition of ICI use is not straightforward, however current recommendations include discontinuation in the context of severe anemia.
- Rechallenging patients with an ICI once the anemia is corrected remains a point of debate and must be discussed within the context of the patient's underlying malignancy and therapeutic options together with oncology.

DISCLOSURES

No conflicts of interest or disclosures to declare.

REFERENCES

1. Saliba AN, Xie Z, Higgins AS, et al. Immune-related hematologic adverse events in the context of immune checkpoint inhibitor therapy. Am J Hematol 2021;96(10). E362-e7.
2. Tanios GE, Doley PB, Munker R. Autoimmune hemolytic anemia associated with the use of immune checkpoint inhibitors for cancer: 68 cases from the Food and Drug Administration database and review. Eur J Haematol 2019;102(2):157–62.
3. June CH, Sadelain M. Chimeric Antigen Receptor Therapy. N Engl J Med 2018; 379(1):64–73.
4. Kiem D, Leisch M, Neureiter D, et al. Two Cases of Pancytopenia with Coombs-Negative Hemolytic Anemia after Chimeric Antigen Receptor T-Cell Therapy. Int J Mol Sci 2021;22(11).
5. Delanoy N, Michot JM, Comont T, et al. Haematological immune-related adverse events induced by anti-PD-1 or anti-PD-L1 immunotherapy: a descriptive observational study. Lancet Haematol 2019;6(1):e48–57.

6. Klein NP, Ray P, Carpenter D, et al. Rates of autoimmune diseases in Kaiser Permanente for use in vaccine adverse event safety studies. Vaccine 2010;28(4): 1062–8.

7. Lechner K, Jäger U. How I treat autoimmune hemolytic anemias in adults. Blood 2010;116(11):1831–8.

8. Gehrs BC, Friedberg RC. Autoimmune hemolytic anemia. Am J Hematol 2002; 69(4):258–71.

9. Eaton WW, Rose NR, Kalaydjian A, et al. Epidemiology of autoimmune diseases in Denmark. J Autoimmun 2007;29(1):1–9.

10. Baek DW, Chae YS. Pembrolizumab-related autoimmune hemolytic anemia in a patient with metastatic lung adenocarcinoma. Yeungnam Univ J Med 2021; 38(4):366–70.

11. Jobson D, McCormack CJ, Hiscutt E, et al. Severe treatment-resistant autoimmune haemolytic anaemia following ipilimumab in a patient with metastatic melanoma and CLL. Leuk Lymphoma 2021;62(4):992–4.

12. Younce CM, Lawton JM, Patel DR. Atezolizumab-induced hemolytic anemia - A case report. J Oncol Pharm Pract 2021;27(4):1026–8.

13. Atiq O, Atiq SO, Atiq ZO, et al. Pembrolizumab-Induced Cold Agglutinin Disease. Am J Case Rep 2020;21:e924283.

14. Hall M, Meti N, Liontos L, et al. Refractory Autoimmune Hemolytic Anemia and Pure Red Cell Aplasia Secondary to Immunotherapy Requiring Prolonged Immunosuppression. JCO Oncol Pract 2020;16(10):699–700.

15. Hwang SR, O'Dowd T, Markovic SN, et al. Recurrent checkpoint inhibitor-induced warm agglutinin autoimmune hemolytic anemia in a patient with metastatic melanoma. Am J Hematol 2020;95(7). E169-e71.

16. Algaze SD, Park W, Harrington TJ, et al. Autoimmune haemolytic anaemia in a patient with advanced lung adenocarcinoma and chronic lymphocytic leukaemia receiving nivolumab and intravenous immunoglobulin. BMJ Case Rep 2018;2018.

17. Hasanov M, Konoplev SN, Hernandez CMR. Nivolumab-induced cold agglutinin syndrome successfully treated with rituximab. Blood Adv 2018;2(15):1865–8.

18. Johnstone P, Khan O. Pembrolizumab-associated autoimmune haemolytic anaemia. BMJ Case Rep 2019;12(10).

19. Khan U, Ali F, Khurram MS, et al. Immunotherapy-associated autoimmune hemolytic anemia. J Immunother Cancer 2017;5:15.

20. Leaf RK, Ferreri C, Rangachari D, et al. Clinical and laboratory features of autoimmune hemolytic anemia associated with immune checkpoint inhibitors. Am J Hematol 2019;94(5):563–74.

21. Ni D, AlZahrani F, Smylie M. AIHA and Pancytopenia as Complications of Pembrolizumab Therapy for Metastatic Melanoma: A Case Report. Case Rep Oncol 2019;12(2):456–65.

22. Ogawa K, Ito J, Fujimoto D, et al. Exacerbation of autoimmune hemolytic anemia induced by the first dose of programmed death-1 inhibitor pembrolizumab: a case report. Invest New Drugs 2018;36(3):509–12.

23. Ramos B, Gastal G, Rovere RK. An Autoimmune Haemolytic Anaemia Secondary to Ipilimumab Treatment. Klin Onkol 2017;30(2):128–30.

24. Shaikh H, Daboul N, Albrethsen M, et al. A case of autoimmune haemolytic anaemia after 39 cycles of nivolumab. BMJ Case Rep 2018;2018.

25. Tardy MP, Gastaud L, Boscagli A, et al. Autoimmune hemolytic anemia after nivolumab treatment in Hodgkin lymphoma responsive to immunosuppressive treatment. A case report. Hematol Oncol 2017;35(4):875–7.

26. Williams H, Aitchison R. Pembrolizumab-induced autoimmune haemolytic anaemia and cholangitis. BMJ Case Rep 2019;12(12).
27. Barcellini W, Fattizzo B. The Changing Landscape of Autoimmune Hemolytic Anemia. Front Immunol 2020;11:946.
28. Karafin MS, Denomme GA, Schanen M, et al. Clinical and reference lab characteristics of patients with suspected direct antiglobulin test (DAT)-negative immune hemolytic anemia. Immunohematology 2015;31(3):108–15.
29. Kramer R, Zaremba A, Moreira A, et al. Hematological immune related adverse events after treatment with immune checkpoint inhibitors. Eur J Cancer 2021;147: 170–81.
30. Worlledge SM. Immune drug-induced haemolytic anemias. Semin Hematol 1969; 6(2):181–200.
31. Barcellini W. New Insights in the Pathogenesis of Autoimmune Hemolytic Anemia. Transfus Med Hemother 2015;42(5):287–93.
32. Go RS, Winters JL, Kay NE. How I treat autoimmune hemolytic anemia. Blood 2017;129(22):2971–9.
33. Arndt PA, Garratty G. The changing spectrum of drug-induced immune hemolytic anemia. Semin Hematol 2005;42(3):137–44.
34. Krummel MF, Allison JP. CTLA-4 engagement inhibits IL-2 accumulation and cell cycle progression upon activation of resting T cells. J Exp Med 1996;183(6):2533–40.
35. Boussiotis VA. Molecular and Biochemical Aspects of the PD-1 Checkpoint Pathway. N Engl J Med 2016;375(18):1767–78.
36. Alsaab HO, Sau S, Alzhrani R, et al. PD-1 and PD-L1 Checkpoint Signaling Inhibition for Cancer Immunotherapy: Mechanism, Combinations, and Clinical Outcome. Front Pharmacol 2017;8:561.
37. Zou W, Chen L. Inhibitory B7-family molecules in the tumour microenvironment. Nat Rev Immunol 2008;8(6):467–77.
38. Jain NA, Zhao S, Wei L, et al. Association Between RBC Antigen Allo-Antibodies and Immune-Related Adverse Events During Immune Checkpoint Inhibitor Treatment for Advanced Cancers. Cancer Manag Res 2020;12:11743–9.
39. Bell CA, Zwicker H, Sacks HJ. Autoimmune hemolytic anemia: routine serologic evaluation in a general hospital population. Am J Clin Pathol 1973;60(6):903–11.
40. Dausset J, Colombani J. The serology and the prognosis of 128 cases of autoimmune hemolytic anemia. Blood 1959;14:1280–301.
41. Sokol RJ, Hewitt S, Stamps BK. Autoimmune haemolysis: an 18-year study of 865 cases referred to a regional transfusion centre. Br Med J (Clin Res Ed 1981; 282(6281):2023–7.
42. Schneider BJ, Naidoo J, Santomasso BD, et al. Management of Immune-Related Adverse Events in Patients Treated With Immune Checkpoint Inhibitor Therapy: ASCO Guideline Update. J Clin Oncol 2021;Jco2101440.
43. Berentsen S, Barcellini W, D'Sa S, et al. Cold agglutinin disease revisited: a multinational, observational study of 232 patients. Blood 2020;136(4):480–8.
44. Murphy S, LoBuglio AF. Drug therapy of autoimmune hemolytic anemia. Semin Hematol 1976;13(4):323–34.
45. Barcellini W, Fattizzo B, Zaninoni A, et al. Clinical heterogeneity and predictors of outcome in primary autoimmune hemolytic anemia: a GIMEMA study of 308 patients. Blood 2014;124(19):2930–6.
46. Jäger U, Barcellini W, Broome CM, et al. Diagnosis and treatment of autoimmune hemolytic anemia in adults: Recommendations from the First International Consensus Meeting. Blood Rev 2020;41:100648.

47. Roumier M, Loustau V, Guillaud C, et al. Characteristics and outcome of warm autoimmune hemolytic anemia in adults: New insights based on a single-center experience with 60 patients. Am J Hematol 2014;89(9):E150–5.
48. Kulpa J, Skrabs C, Simanek R, et al. Probability of remaining in unsustained complete remission after steroid therapy withdrawal in patients with primary warm-antibody reactive autoimmune hemolytic anemia. Wien Klin Wochenschr 2016; 128(7–8):234–7.
49. Flores G, Cunningham-Rundles C, Newland AC, et al. Efficacy of intravenous immunoglobulin in the treatment of autoimmune hemolytic anemia: results in 73 patients. Am J Hematol 1993;44(4):237–42.
50. Costa RH, Draper KG, Kelly TJ, et al. An unusual spliced herpes simplex virus type 1 transcript with sequence homology to Epstein-Barr virus DNA. J Virol 1985;54(2):317–28.
51. Patel NY, Chilsen AM, Mathiason MA, et al. Outcomes and complications after splenectomy for hematologic disorders. Am J Surg 2012;204(6):1014–9.
52. Balagué C, Targarona EM, Cerdán G, et al. Long-term outcome after laparoscopic splenectomy related to hematologic diagnosis. Surg Endosc 2004; 18(8):1283–7.
53. Dierickx D, Kentos A, Delannoy A. The role of rituximab in adults with warm antibody autoimmune hemolytic anemia. Blood 2015;125(21):3223–9.
54. Hill QA, Stamps R, Massey E, et al. Guidelines on the management of drug-induced immune and secondary autoimmune, haemolytic anaemia. Br J Haematol 2017;177(2):208–20.
55. Bussone G, Ribeiro E, Dechartres A, et al. Efficacy and safety of rituximab in adults' warm antibody autoimmune haemolytic anemia: retrospective analysis of 27 cases. Am J Hematol 2009;84(3):153–7.
56. Maung SW, Leahy M, O'Leary HM, et al. A multi-centre retrospective study of rituximab use in the treatment of relapsed or resistant warm autoimmune haemolytic anaemia. Br J Haematol 2013;163(1):118–22.
57. Birgens H, Frederiksen H, Hasselbalch HC, et al. A phase III randomized trial comparing glucocorticoid monotherapy versus glucocorticoid and rituximab in patients with autoimmune haemolytic anaemia. Br J Haematol 2013;163(3): 393–9.
58. Michel M, Terriou L, Roudot-Thoraval F, et al. A randomized and double-blind controlled trial evaluating the safety and efficacy of rituximab for warm autoimmune hemolytic anemia in adults (the RAIHA study). Am J Hematol 2017; 92(1):23–7.
59. Emilia G, Messora C, Longo G, et al. Long-term salvage treatment by cyclosporin in refractory autoimmune haematological disorders. Br J Haematol 1996;93(2): 341–4.
60. Moyo VM, Smith D, Brodsky I, et al. High-dose cyclophosphamide for refractory autoimmune hemolytic anemia. Blood 2002;100(2):704–6.
61. Howard J, Hoffbrand AV, Prentice HG, et al. Mycophenolate mofetil for the treatment of refractory auto-immune haemolytic anaemia and auto-immune thrombocytopenia purpura. Br J Haematol 2002;117(3):712–5.
62. Barcellini W, Zaninoni A, Fattizzo B, et al. Predictors of refractoriness to therapy and healthcare resource utilization in 378 patients with primary autoimmune hemolytic anemia from eight Italian reference centers. Am J Hematol 2018;93(9). E243-e6.
63. Barcellini W, Fattizzo B, Zaninoni A. Current and emerging treatment options for autoimmune hemolytic anemia. Expert Rev Clin Immunol 2018;14(10):857–72.

64. Barcellini W, Zaninoni A, Giannotta JA, et al. New Insights in Autoimmune Hemolytic Anemia: From Pathogenesis to Therapy Stage 1. J Clin Med 2020;9(12).
65. Berentsen S, Ulvestad E, Langholm R, et al. Primary chronic cold agglutinin disease: a population based clinical study of 86 patients. Haematologica 2006; 91(4):460–6.
66. Jaffe CJ, Atkinson JP, Frank MM. The role of complement in the clearance of cold agglutinin-sensitized erythrocytes in man. J Clin Invest 1976;58(4):942–9.
67. Nydegger UE, Kazatchkine MD, Miescher PA. Immunopathologic and clinical features of hemolytic anemia due to cold agglutinins. Semin Hematol 1991; 28(1):66–77.
68. Schöllkopf C, Kjeldsen L, Bjerrum OW, et al. Rituximab in chronic cold agglutinin disease: a prospective study of 20 patients. Leuk Lymphoma 2006;47(2):253–60.
69. Berentsen S, Ulvestad E, Gjertsen BT, et al. Rituximab for primary chronic cold agglutinin disease: a prospective study of 37 courses of therapy in 27 patients. Blood 2004;103(8):2925–8.
70. Berentsen S, Randen U, Oksman M, et al. Bendamustine plus rituximab for chronic cold agglutinin disease: results of a Nordic prospective multicenter trial. Blood 2017;130(4):537–41.
71. Pollack MH, Betof A, Dearden H, et al. Safety of resuming anti-PD-1 in patients with immune-related adverse events (irAEs) during combined anti-CTLA-4 and anti-PD1 in metastatic melanoma. Ann Oncol 2018;29(1):250–5.

Adult Evans' Syndrome

Marc Michel, MD, MSc

KEYWORDS

- Evans syndrome • Autoimmune cytopenia • Autoimmune hemolytic anemia
- Immune thrombocytopenic purpura • Autoimmune neutropenia
- Primary immunodeficiencies

KEY POINTS

- The differential diagnosis of Evans syndrome includes thrombotic thrombocytopenic purpura and the analysis of the blood smear is very important.
- Evans syndrome during childhood is frequently associated with an inborn error or immunity.
- Secondary cases of Evans syndrome in adults represent 20% to 50% of all cases.
- Rituximab is the best second-line treatment option for adult onset Evans syndrome.

DEFINITION AND EPIDEMIOLOGY

Evans syndrome (ES) which was first described by Evans in 1951[1] is a rare auto-immune disease defined as the concomitant or sequential occurrence of immune thrombocytopenia (ITP) and warm autoimmune haemolytic anemia (wAIHA) ± autoimmune neutropenia (AIN) which is present in about 20% of the patients.[2] Autoimmune cytopenias (AIC) may occur either simultaneously in 30% to 50% of the cases[2,3] or sequentially with a mean delay between both cytopenias of 3 years,[4] ITP preceding wAIHA in about a third of the cases %.[2,3] The 3 cytopenias occur concomitantly in only 10% of the cases.[3] The mean delay between the different AIC is of 3 years, but is highly variable.[3,4] ES can be either isolated and defined as primary or secondary if associated with an underlying disease.[3] As for wAIHA,[5] the rate of secondary ES is known varies from 20% to 50% based on the data from the literature.[2,3] Underlying associated conditions are mostly represented by lymphoproliferative disorders (LPD) and systemic lupus erythematosus (SLE) in adults,[2,3] whereas ES in children often reveals and underlying primary immunodeficiency/inborn errors of immunity.[6]

In a recent Danish nationwide epidemiologic study focused on ES, mean age at diagnosis was 58.5 years at diagnosis[7] in keeping with a previous report of 68 adults

Department of Internal Medicine, National Referral Center for Adult Immune Cytopenias Henri Mondor University Hospital, Service de Medecine Interne, CHU Hopital Henri-Mondor, Assistance Publique Hôpitaux de Paris, Université Paris-Est Créteil, 51 Av du Mal de Lattre de Tassigny, 94010 Creteil Cedex, France
E-mail address: marc.michel2@aphp.fr

Hematol Oncol Clin N Am 36 (2022) 381–392
https://doi.org/10.1016/j.hoc.2021.12.004
0889-8588/22/© 2021 Elsevier Inc. All rights reserved.

with ES,[3] sex ratio was close to 1 (51.2% of women), whereas only 27.3% of the cases were classified as secondary. The annual estimated incidence of ES in Denmark was 1.8 per million person-years with a prevalence of 21.30 per million individuals.[7] When considering isolated AIC, ES represents 0.3% to 7% of AIHA and approximately 2% to 2.7% of all ITP cases.[3,7,8]

DIAGNOSIS OF EVANS SYNDROME

When ITP and wAIHA occur sequentially, each AIC is diagnosed based on usual criteria[5,9] and the diagnosis of ES is considered when the second AIC occurs. As a reminder, the diagnosis of ITP is one of the exclusion in the presence of isolated thrombocytopenia (platelet count <100 × 10^9/L)[9] while the diagnosis of wAIHA implies not only the presence of a newly diagnosed hemolytic anemia but also the positivity of the direct antiglobulin test (DAT) with an IgG or IgG + C3d pattern.[5] When both cytopenias and pancytopenia occur simultaneously in a patient with no previous medical history the diagnosis may be more difficult and some differential diagnosis must be ruled out. Patients with ES may clinically present with both nonspecific symptoms of hemolytic anemia (fatigue, exertional dyspnea, jaundice ± dark urine) and/or bleeding manifestations including petechiae, spontaneous bruises ± gum bleeding and oral bullae and/or epistaxis in case of profound thrombocytopenia. Mild splenomegaly is present at onset in approximately 1/3 of the patients[2] especially in the case of active wAIHA. It must be emphasized that no organ dysfunction/failure, headache, or fever are usually observed in patients with ES except in the very rare event of intracranial hemorrhage. In the presence of concomitant thrombocytopenia and hemolytic anemia, the first step of the diagnostic procedure is to check both the renal function and the peripheral blood smear.[4] In typical ES, renal function is normal and there are no or very few schistocytes on the smear and as for isolated wAIHA, some spherocytes can be observed.[10] The presence of spherocytes reflect the partial phagocytosis of autologous RBCs opsonized by autoantibodies.[5] Another common feature seen on the blood smear in ES being poikilocytosis. In the presence of numerous schistocytes (>10% of RBCs), the diagnosis of thrombotic microangiopathy (TMA) and especially thrombotic thrombocytopenic purpura (TTP) must be suspected. When schistocytes are initially absent or present in a low number and the diagnosis is not obvious, the assessment of schistocytes on blood smear must be repeated over a few days and the diagnoses of ES should be promptly reconsidered especially when first-line treatments are ineffective.[11] When clinical and biological features of TMA are present, based on the French score and/or the PLASMIC score, the presence or absence of organ damage, the level of serum creatinine and the severity of thrombocytopenia are particularly helpful for distinguishing between typical or atypical hemolytic uremic syndrome (HUS) and TTP.[12] When ES occurs during pregnancy[13] and especially at the 3rd trimester other diagnosis such as HELLP (Hemolysis with Elevated Liver enzymes and Low Platelet count) syndrome and preeclampsia must be ruled out. Another diagnosis that may mimic TTP and ES is catastrophic antiphospholipid syndrome (CAPS).[14] The distinguishing features between ES, TTP, and CAPS entities are summarized in **Table 1**. Of note, patients with an underlying SLE are particularly at risk of developing such complications and they have a positive DAT at baseline and develop TTP or CAPS rather than ES.[14,15]

Among other differential diagnoses of ES, marked macrocytic anemia with markers of hemolysis (ie, high LDH level due to ineffective erythropoiesis in the marrow) and mild thrombocytopenia with the presence of numerous schistocytes on the blood smear may also rarely reveal vitamin B12 deficiency.[16] The high level of the mean

Table 1
Distinguishing clinical and biological features between Evans syndrome, acquired autoimmune thrombotic thrombocytopenic purpura, and CAPS

	Evans Syndrome	Acquired Thrombotic Thrombocytopenic Purpura (aTTP)	Catastrophic Antiphospholipid Syndrome (CAPS)
Patient's profile: gender, mean age	Women (60%), 55 y	Women (70%), 40–45 y	Women (70%), 35 y, Underlying SLE (40%)
Organ failure	NO	YES + (kidney, central nervous system, heart)	YES ++ by definition (kidney, central nervous system, hear, lung)
Platelet count <30 × 10⁹/L Severity of hemolytic anemia	Frequent mild to severe (can be life-threatening)	Frequent mild	Rare mild
Bleeding manifestations	Frequent and sometimes severe when the platelet count is <20 × 10⁹/L	Absent or mild	Absent ou minor
Acute renal insufficiency	Absent	Minimal to mild	Mild to severe
Severe hypertension	NO	NO	Frequent
Schizocyte on the blood smear	Absents of few	+ to +++	++
Direct antiglobulin test	Strongly positive in ∼ 95% of the cases	Rarely weakly positive (10%–15%)	Usually negative, rarely weekly +
ADAMTS13 activity	Normal	≤ 10%	Normal or mildly decreased

Abbreviations: ADAMTS, a disintegrin and metalloproteinase with thrombospondin type 1 motifs; member, 13; SLE, systemic lupus erythematosus.

corpuscular volume (MCV) associated with a normal reticulocyte count and the absence of organ failure and bleeding manifestations make this hypothesis more likely than TTP of ES.[16]

The next step of the diagnostic procedure is based on the result of the DAT which is classically strongly positive, mostly with an IgG or IgG + C3d pattern in 85% of the cases in keeping with wAIHA.[2] About 5% of patients with ES may have a mixed AIHA subtype or even (∼5% of the case) a DAT that is only C3d positive with the presence of cold agglutinins at a significant titer.[2] As for isolated AIHA, the DAT may be negative in about 5% of the cases in ES and in that such other causes of acquired of hemolytic anemia such as paroxysmal nocturnal hemoglobinuria (PNH) must be ruled out, and a PNH clone must be looked for by means of flow cytometry.[17] On the other hand, the DAT may be weekly positive in definite cases of TTP and that can be a source of misdiagnosis which can be avoided by testing rapidly ADAMTS13 activity which is by definition constantly strongly decreased (≤10%) in TTP.[11] Overall, the absence of schistocytes on the blood smear and a strongly positive DAT in a patient that has not received recently a transfusion of packed red cells makes the diagnosis of ES very likely. **Table 1** summarizes the main distinguishing features between ES, TTP, and CAPS at the time of disease onset.

Most of the time, when ITP and wAIHA occur concomitantly with typical features of hemolysis are present and reticulocytosis (ie, reticulocytes count >120 $\times$ 10^9/L), there is no need to systematically perform a marrow aspirate ($\pm$karyotype) or biopsy for confirming ES. Conversely, when ES presents only with ITP and AIN or if there are some atypical features (atypical lymphocytes, pseudo-Pelger–Huët anomalies...) on the smear and an LPD with a concomitant bone marrow involvement or an associated myelodysplastic syndrome is suspected, performing a marrow analysis is relevant.[4,5] An s for primary ITP, there is usually no need to look for the presence of antiplatelet antibodies by means of MAIPA (monoclonal antibody-specific immobilization of platelet antigen) in ES when other common causes of thrombocytopenia (liver disease, TMA, coagulopathy...) have been excluded as their specificity is not optimal and the sensitivity of the assay is rather low.[9] When neutropenia is present in combination with thrombocytopenia and/or hemolytic anemia in the setting of ES, there is no consensus about the utility of searching for the presence of antibodies directed toward neutrophils by means of MAIGA (monoclonal antibody-specific immobilization of platelet antigen).[18]

PRIMARY OR SECONDARY EVANS SYNDROME

Once the diagnosis of ES is confirmed and an appropriate treatment has been initiated, the next step of the diagnostic procedure is to search for an underlying disease or condition that may influence both the treatment and the outcome of ES.[4] The occurrence of several AIC in a single patient reflects an important immune dysregulation toward self-antigens and the rate of secondary ES may vary from 20% to more than 50% according to the age population and the intensity of the workup that is performed at the time of disease onset.[2,3,19]

The main causes of secondary ES are summarized in **Box 1**. In children and adolescents, primary immunodeficiencies (PID), now most often renamed human inborn errors of immunity or IEIs,[20] are by far the most frequent causes of ES.[7,21] Common variable immunodeficiency (CVID) is known to be associated with an increased risk of autoimmunity and especially of immune cytopenias including ES[7,22] and, as for primary ITP and wAIHA, checking the level of gammaglobulin in the serum in every child diagnosed with ES before using intravenous immunoglobulin (IVIg) has become a standard and a good practice. The reasons why patients with hypogammaglobulinemia in the setting of CVID or other IEIs are at high risk of autoimmunity and especially of immune cytopenias are far from being fully understood.[23] Autoimmune lymphoproliferative syndrome (ALPS) is also known to cause ES[24] and looking for the presence of excess (>5%) TCR$\alpha\beta^+$ CD3$^+$ CD4$^-$/CD8$^-$ double-negative T cells at disease onset should, therefore, be standard of care in children diagnosed with ES, ideally before the use of high dose of corticosteroids. In the last decade, the extended use of next-generation sequencing (NGS) and whole exome sequencing (WES) has led to the discovery and description of several new genetic defects that may be associated with an increased risk of ES such as CTLA4 (cytotoxic T-lymphocyte-associated protein 4) and LRBA (LPS Responsive Beige-Like Anchor Protein) defects or SOCS1 (suppressor of cytokine signaling 1) haploinsufficiency.[6,25] It is, therefore, very important that physicians who are involved in the management of pediatric ES be aware of the need of looking for possible consanguinity and/or a history of AIC, LPD among relatives throughout a family tree.

Box 1
Main disorders or conditions associated with Evans' syndrome (secondary cases)

1. Lymphoproliferative diseases and other hematologic diseases:
   a. Chronic lymphoid leukemia T-cell LGL leukemia
   b. B-cell lymphoma/Hodgkin lymphoma
   c. Angioimmunoblastic T cell lymphoma
   d. Castleman disease
   e. Chronic myelomonocytic leukemia

2. *Solid tumors*: Thymoma/ovarian dermoid cyst/carcinoma

3. Auto-immune and inflammatory diseases
   a. Systemic lupus erythematosus/Antiphospholipid syndrome
   b. The connective tissue diseases
   c. Ulcerative colitis/Crohn's disease

4. Infections:
   Virus: Ebstein Barr virus/hepatitis C/cytomegalovirus, SARS-CoV-2

5. *Drugs*: checkpoint inhibitors (anti-PD1: nivolumab)

6. Primary immunodeficiencies/inborn errors of immunity
   a. Common variable immunodeficiency
   b. Hyper IgM syndrome[a]/ALPS[a]
   c. CTLA4 deficiency[a], LRBA deficiency[a], SOCS1 haploinsufficiency[a]
   d. IPEX syndrome[a]/APECED syndrome[a]

7. Others:
   a. Postallogenic bone marrow transplantation
   b. Pregnancy
   c. Kabuki syndrome[a]

Abbreviations: ALPS, Autoimmune lymphoproliferative syndrome; APECED, Autoimmune poly-endocrinopathy with candidiasis and ectodermal dystrophy; IPEX, immune dysregulation, Pol-yendocrinopathy; Enteropathy X-linked; LGL, large granular lymphocytes.

[a] Almost exclusively diagnosed revealed by ES during childhood or adolescence.

While the diagnosis of ALPS in young adults is possible,[24] CVID is by far the most frequent PID diagnosed in adulthood.[22] Regarding LPDs, B-cell lymphomas, and especially chronic lymphocytic leukemia (CLL) are the most frequent causes of ES[26–28] and therefore, immunophenotyping of B cells should be performed in every adult patient diagnosed with ES and lymphoma must be suspected in a patient with ES and disproportionate splenomegaly and/or lymph nodes. ES has been reported in up to 2.9% in a cohort of patients with CLL. In half of the cases, autoimmune cytopenias occurred simultaneously and revealed CLL in 25% of cases.[27] The median age at ES diagnosis was 66 years and 60% of patients were male. Although there was no difference regarding demographic or Binet stage between patients with or without ES; patient with CLL-associated ES had more frequently immunologic and/or genetic markers of poor prognosis at CLL diagnosis, such as a higher expression of ZAP-70, an increase in unmutated IGHV, del (17) or TP53 mutation leading to the reduction of their overall survival.[27] While other types of B cell lymphoma[28] or T-cell lymphoma[29] may seldom be associated with ES, occurrence of ES in patients with a history of Hodgkin lymphoma is very rare unless they had autologous stem cell transplantation.[4]

Another classical cause of ES in adults is SLE[3,10] and therefore, searching for the presence of positive antinuclear antibodies should be systematic at the time of ES. Regarding infections that may trigger ES, SARS-CoV-2 has been recently recognized as a potential cause of ES.[30] Drug-induced ES is excessively rare but the increased use of checkpoint inhibitors in oncology and especially the anti-PD1 nivolumab has been associated with an increased risk of ITP/AIHA that may seldom occur concomitantly.[31] There is no consensus about the workup that should be performed in every patient with ES to look for an underlying cause and the need for a systematic bone marrow aspirate or biopsy is a matter of debate as up to 39% of the patients displayed features of underlying myelodysplasia in the recent series from Fatizzo and colleagues.[2] By analogy with the one recommended for wAIHA,[5] a proposal of workup for ES is provided in **Table 2**. Although the onset of ES may sometimes precede by many months or years the occurrence of an LPD[28] or SLE,[32] there are no specific recommendations about the necessity of repeating the initial workup at regular intervals during follow-up.

MANAGEMENT OF ADULT EVANS SYNDROME

ES runs a chronic course (>1 year) in more than 80% of the cases, with multiple relapses.[2,4] Despite continuous progress in the management of AIC and a gradual increase in ES survival, the mortality due to ES which is 20% to 24%[2,3] remains higher than the ones of isolated AIC, the main causes of deaths being infections,

Table 2
Recommendations for the diagnosis of secondary Evans syndrome in adults

Disease or Condition	Tests to be Performed Systematically	Tests to be Considered Only in Some Circumstances
SLE and other autoimmune diseases	• **Antinuclear Abs (ANA)** and if + with titer >1/80: anti-dsDNA Abs and other specificities	• Lupus anticoagulant • Anticardiolipin Abs • Anti-β2gpI Abs (only for patients with overt SLE, strongly positive ANA or past history of thrombosis) • CH50, C3, and C4 in case of SLE
Lymphoproliferative disorders and solid tumors	• **Blood smear** (increase rate of LGL?) • **Serum protein electrophoresis** • **Immunoelectrophoresis** • **Immunophenotyping of B lymphocytes** from peripheral blood • [a]**CT scan** (chest/abdomen/pelvis)	• Bone marrow biopsy ≥especially in the presence of monoclonal gammopathy or hypogammaglobulinemia and/or lymph nodes and/or disproportionate splenomegaly on the CT scan and/or monotypic lymphocytes population • Lymph node biopsy • TEP-scan
Primary immunodeficiency	• **IgG, IgA and IgM levels**	• Extended phenotype of T/NK and memory B cells • Postvaccine (eg, tetanus toxoid, pneumococcal) serologies
Infections	• **HIV, HCV, and (HBV)[b] tests**	• CMV, EBV, Parvovirus B19, SARS-CoV-2, and others based on clinical and/or biological evidence

Abbreviations: Abs, antibodies; ds, double strand; LGL, large granular lymphocytes; SLE, systemic lupus erythematosus.
[a] Unless diagnosis of SLE is obvious.
[b] Mostly pretherapeutic.

thromboembolic events and bleeding and the main predictor of mortality in adults is the severity of AIHA at diagnosis[2,3]

Primary Evans syndrome

The management of patients with ES is mainly extrapolated from the one of the ITP and wAIHA or based on retrospective case series and when both cytopenias occur sequentially, they are treated as single cytopenias according to consensual recommendations of guidelines.[5,9] When both cytopenias occur concomitantly in the setting of primary ES, treatment is most often indicated as spontaneous remissions or durable compensated hemolysis with a stable Hb level above 10 g/dL is very uncommon.[5] Corticosteroids remain the cornerstone of first-line treatment predniso(lo)ne at the initial daily dose of 1 mg/kg is the standard of care. The efficacy of repeated courses of dexamethasone toward predniso(lo)ne has not been specifically tested in ES, but based on the data available in ITP,[33] it can be viewed as a relevant alternative. In case of severe bleeding manifestations, the use of IVIg at a dose of 1 to 2 g/kg in combination with corticosteroids is required to avoid a life-threatening hemorrhage,[9] whereas IVIg has only a little efficacy for the management of severe wAIHA.[34] For patients with severe wAIHA, transfusion, or packed RBCs must not be postponed,[35] and the transient use of recombinant erythropoietin may be useful for those patients with severe wAIHA an inadequate reticulocytosis.[36] Predniso(lo)ne is usually maintained at the initial dose for 3 weeks followed by progressive weaning over at least a 3 months as usually recommended for adult wAIHA.[5] For patients not responding to predniso(lo)ne, the daily dose can be transiently increased up to a maximum of 2 mg/kg, although the efficacy of such a dose has never been fully demonstrated. Most of the patients ($\sim$80%) have an initial response, but the time to response and the magnitude of response on the platelet count on one side and hemoglobin levels and parameters of hemolysis in the other side, may be significantly different, and differential patterns of response are not uncommon.[3] In the absence of initial response ($\sim$20% of the patients), or in case of corticosteroid-dependency with the need of maintaining a daily dose of predniso(lo)ne of more than 10 mg to maintain at least a partial response (ie, a platelet count $\geq$30 $\times$ 10^9/L with at least a doubling of the initial count and/or a Hb level $\geq$10 g/dL with a least a 2 g increase from baseline), a second-line therapy is needed. Overall, 60% to 76% of adult with ES require a second line.[2] Although rituximab is not licensed for ITP and/or AIHA, its efficacy and good safety profile have been shown throughout randomized prospective studies.[36–38] To a lesser extent, the efficacy of rituximab has only be reported in both adult and pediatric ES based on retrospective studies[2,3,39] with an overall response rate (ORR) reaching up 96% in some series.[2] For patients not responding to rituximab, the 3rd treatment-line option can be either the use of an immunosuppressant such as azathioprine, cyclosporin or mycophenolate mofetil or yet splenectomy.[2–4] There is not enough data available in ES for recommending a specific immunosuppressant, and the choice mostly relies on the expected risk over benefit ratio on an individual basis as well as on the experience of the treating physician. The ORR with splenectomy varies from 52% to 100% according to the series from the literature[2,3,40] and for ES not responding to rituximab with the sustained activity of both itp and wAIHA, splenectomy definitely remains a good option. When only itp remains active and symptomatic after corticosteroids $\pm$ rituximab, the use of a thrombopoietin receptor agonist (Tpo-RA) such as eltrombopag or romiplostim is relevant and effective.[2] For patients with multi-refractory ES, targeting long-lived autoreactive plasma cells by means of bortezomib combined with dexamethasone[41,42] or daratumumab[43] may be a good option. Another option in the future could also be to use fostamatinib, a spleen tyrosine kinase (*syk*) inhibitor that has been approved for adult' primary ITP and that has also shown a promising efficacy for wAIHA in a phase II trial.[44] Other treatment approaches currently developed in both ITP and wAIHA such as FcRn or complement inhibitors could also find a place in the future for the treatment of ES. An algorithm for the management of primary adult ES is provided in **Fig. 1**.

Secondary Evans syndrome

The management of patients with secondary ES must take into account the nature and activity of the underlying/associated disorder. For SLE or CVID-associated ES, the initial strategy is similar to the one of the primary ES, rituximab being a good corticosteroid-sparing 2nd line option[45,46] while splenectomy is not recommended in those settings. If ES occurs in patient with an underlying active SLE with a previous or concomitant history of lupus nephritis, the use of mycophenolate mofetil in combination with prednisone is more relevant.[32] When rituximab is given for treating a patient with ES who has an underlying CVID, replacement therapy with subcutaneous Ig must be systematic to avoid severe infections.[46] Moreover, Tpo-RAs should be used with caution in patients with SLE or APS-associated ES and active itp as there is in increased risk of thrombosis in that setting.[47] For patients with CLL or lymphoma-associated ES, the management of ES must obviously take into account the activity and stage of clonal LPD[27,28] and some regimens combining for example, rituximab + cyclophosphamide and dexamethasone can be helpful for treating CLL-associated ES.[48] For young patients with ALPS, sirolimus may be a good option,[49] whereas splenectomy must be avoided as the risk of overwhelming postsplenectomy infections is very high in this patient population.

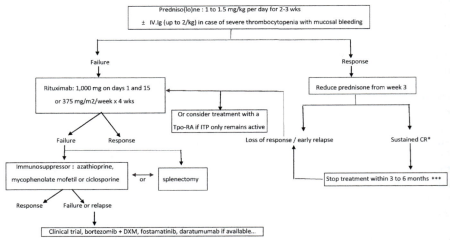

Fig. 1. Proposed algorithm for the treatment of *primary* * *Evans syndrome* with concomitant AIHA and ITP ± AIN in adults. *Excluding especially patients with an underlying lymphoma or with some immunodeficiencies for which rituximab and/or splenectomy may be contra-indicated; ** Complete response = Hemoglobin level greater than 12 g/dL without ongoing hemolysis and platelet count $\geq$ 100 × 10^9/L; *** if a daily dose of predni(solo)ne $\leq$ 10 mg is sufficient to maintain the hemoglobin level above 10 g/dL and the platelet count greater than 30 × 10^9/L, it can be maintained on a long-term.

SUMMARY

Evans syndrome is a very rare autoimmune condition reflecting a major breakdown of immune self-tolerance. ES can be life-threatening with an overall mortality rate of approximately 20% and it is associated with a high rate of severe infections and thrombosis. The diagnosis of ES may be difficult and requires a minimal initial workup to rule-out some other diagnoses of bi-cytopenia (ie, thrombocytopenia + hemolytic anemia) and mostly thrombotic microangiopathies. The rate of secondary ES varies from 20 to up to 50% among adults and searching accurately for an underlying disease at the time of diagnosis is important as it may have an impact on both the prognosis and management. The management of ES is mostly extrapolated from the standard of care of both ITP and wAIHA which is currently rapidly evolving. An increasing number of inborn errors of immunity have been described in the last decade especially among children or adolescents with ES, and these new insights are helpful for a better comprehension of the pathophysiology of ES also in adults and preclude the use of more targeted therapies in the future.

REFERENCES

1. Evans RS, Takahashi K, Duane RT, et al. Primary thrombocytopenic purpura and acquired hemolytic anemia; evidence for a common etiology. AMA Arch Intern Med 1951;87:48–65.
2. Fattizzo B, Michel M, Giannotta JA, et al. Evans syndrome in adults: an observational multicentre study. Blood Adv 2021;5(24):5468–78.
3. Michel M, Chanet V, Dechartres A, et al. The spectrum of Evans syndrome in adults: new insight into the disease based on the analysis of 68 cases. Blood 2009;114:3167–72.
4. Audia S, Grienay N, Mounier M, et al. Evans' syndrome: from diagnosis to treatment. J Clin Med 2020;9(12):3851.
5. Jager U, Barcellini W, Broome CM, et al. Diagnosis and treatment of autoimmune hemolytic anemia in adults: recommendations from the first international consensus meeting. Blood Rev 2020;41:16648.
6. Hadjadj J, Aladjidi N, Fernandes H, et al. Pediatric Evans syndrome is associated with a high frequency of potentially damaging variants in immune genes. Blood 2019;134:9–21.
7. Hansen DL, Moller S, Andersen K, et al. Evans syndrome in adults - incidence, prevalence, and survival in a nationwide cohort. Am J Hematol 2019;94:1081–90.
8. Barcellini W, Fattizzo B, Zaninoni A, et al. Clinical heterogeneity and predictors of outcome in primary autoimmune hemolytic anemia: a GIMEMA study of 308 patients. Blood 2014;124:2930–6.
9. Provan D, Arnold DM, Bussel JB, et al. Updated international consensus report on the investigation and management of primary immune thrombocytopenia. Blood Adv 2019;3:3780–817.
10. Roumier M, Loustau V, Guillaud C, et al. Characteristics and outcome of warm autoimmune hemolytic anemia in adults: new insights based on a single-center experience with 60 patients. Am J Hematol 2014;89:E150–5.
11. Grall M, Azoulay E, Galicier L, et al. Thrombotic thrombocytopenic purpura misdiagnosed as autoimmune cytopenia: causes of diagnostic errors and consequence on outcome. Experience of the French thrombotic microangiopathies reference centre. Am J Hematol 2017;92:381–7.
12. Coppo P, Schwarzinger M, Buffet M, et al. French reference center for thrombotic microangiopathies. Predictive features of severe acquired ADAMTS13 deficiency

in idiopathic thrombotic microangiopathies: the French TMA reference center experience. PLoS One 2010;5:e10208.

13. Lefkou E, Nelson-Piercy C, Hunt BJ. Evans' syndrome in pregnancy: a systematic literature review and two new cases. Eur J Obstet Gynecol Reprod Biol 2010; 149:10–7.

14. Cervera R, Rodríguez-Pintó I, Espinosa G. The diagnosis and clinical management of the catastrophic antiphospholipid syndrome: a comprehensive review. J Autoimmun 2018;92:1–11.

15. Lansigan F, Isufi I, Tagoe CE. Microangiopathic haemolytic anaemia resembling thrombotic thrombocytopenic purpura in systemic lupus erythematosus: the role of ADAMTS13. Rheumatology (Oxford) 2011;50(5):824–9.

16. Andres E, Affenberger S, Zimmer J, et al. Current hematological findings in cobalamin deficiency. A study of 201 consecutive patients with documented cobalamin deficiency. Clin Lab Haematol 2006;28:50–6.

17. Brodsky RA. Paroxysmal nocturnal hemoglobinuria. Blood 2014;124:2804–11.

18. Youinou P, Jamin C, Le Pottier L, et al. Diagnostic criteria for autoimmune neutropenia. Autoimmun Rev 2014;13:574–6.

19. Pincez T, Fernandes H, Leblanc T, et al. Long term follow-up of pediatric-onset Evans syndrome: broad immunopathological manifestations and high treatment burden. Haematologica 2021. https://doi.org/10.3324/haematol.2020.27110.

20. Bousfiha A, Jeddane L, Picard C, et al. Human inborn errors of immunity: 2019 update of the IUIS phenotypical classification. J Clin Immunol 2020;40(1):66–81.

21. Besnard C, Levy E, Aladjidi N, et al. Pediatric-onset Evans syndrome: heterogeneous presentation and high frequency of monogenic disorders including LRBA and CTLA4 mutations. Clin Immunol 2018;188:52–7.

22. Feuille EJ, Anooshiravani N, Sullivan KE, et al. Autoimmune cytopenias and associated conditions in CVID: a report from the USIDNET registry. J Clin Immunol 2018;38:28–34.

23. Schmidt RE, Grimbacher B, Witte T. Autoimmunity and primary immunodeficiency: two sides of the same coin? Nat Rev Rheumatol 2017;14(1):7–18.

24. Neven B, Magerus-Chatinet A, Florkin B, et al. A survey of 90 patients with autoimmune lymphoproliferative syndrome related to TNFRSF6 mutation. Blood 2011; 118:4798–807.

25. Hadjadj J, Castro CN, Tusseau M, et al. Early-onset autoimmunity associated with SOCS1 haploinsufficiency. Nat Commun 2020;11(1):5341.

26. Fattizzo B, Barcellini W. Autoimmune cytopenias in chronic lymphocytic leukemia: focus on molecular aspects. Front Oncol 2019;9:1435.

27. Carli G, Visco C, Falisi E, et al. Evans syndrome secondary to chronic lymphocytic leukaemia: presentation, treatment, and outcome. Ann Hematol 2016;95: 863–70.

28. Hauswirth AW, Skrabs C, Schützinger C, et al. Autoimmune hemolytic anemias, Evans' syndromes, and pure red cell aplasia in non-Hodgkin lymphomas. Leuk Lymphoma 2007;48(6):1139–49.

29. Motta G, Vianello F, Menin C, et al. Hepatosplenic gammadelta T-cell lymphoma presenting with immune-mediated thrombocytopenia and hemolytic anemia (Evans' syndrome). Am J Hematol 2002;69(4):272–6.

30. Georgy JT, Jayakaran JAJ, Jacob AS, et al. Evans syndrome and immune thrombocytopenia in two patients with COVID-19. J Med Virol 2021;93(5):2642–4.

31. Delanoy N, Michot JM, Comont T, et al. Haematological immune-related adverse events induced by anti-PD-1 or anti-PD-L1 immunotherapy: a descriptive observational study. Lancet Haematol 2019;6(1):e48–57.

32. Zhang L, Wu X, Wang L, et al. Clinical features of systemic lupus erythematosus patients complicated with Evans syndrome: a case-control, single center study. Medicine 2016;95:e3279.

33. Mithoowani S, Gregory-Miller K, Goy J, et al. High-dose dexamethasone compared with prednisone for previously untreated primary immune thrombocytopenia: a systematic review and meta-analysis. Lancet Haematol 2016;3(10): e489–96.

34. Flores G, Cunningham-Rundles C, Newland AC, et al. Efficacy of intravenous immunoglobulin in the treatment of autoimmune hemolytic anemia: results in 73 patients. Am J Hematol 1993;44:237–42.

35. Buetens OW, Ness PM. Red blood cell transfusion in autoimmune hemolytic anemia. Curr Opin Hematol 2003;10:429–33.

36. Gudbrandsdottir S, Birgens HS, Frederiksen H, et al. Rituximab and dexamethasone vs dexamethasone monotherapy in newly diagnosed patients with primary immune thrombocytopenia. Blood 2013;121:1976–81.

37. Michel M, Terriou L, Roudot-Thoraval F, et al. A randomized and double-blind controlled trial evaluating the safety and efficacy of rituximab for warm autoimmune hemolytic anemia in adults (the RAIHA study). Am J Hematol 2016. https://doi.org/10.1002/ajh.24570.

38. Birgens H, Frederiksen H, Hasselbalch HC, et al. A phase III randomized trial comparing glucocorticoid monotherapy versus glucocorticoid and rituximab in patients with autoimmune haemolytic anaemia. Br J Haematol 2013;163: 393–9.

39. Bader-Meunier B, Aladjidi N, Bellmann F, et al. Rituximab therapy for childhood Evans syndrome. Haematologica 2007;92(12):1691–4.

40. Sulpizio ED, Raghunathan V, Shatzel JJ, et al. Long-term remission rates after splenectomy in adults with Evans syndrome compared to immune thrombocytopenia: a single-center retrospective study. Eur J Haematol 2020;104(1):55–8.

41. Fadlallah J, Michel M, Crickx E, et al. Bortezomib and dexamethasone, an original approach for treating multi-refractory warm autoimmune haemolytic anaemia. Br J Haematol 2019;187(1):124–8.

42. Pasquale R, Giannotta JA, Barcellini W, et al. Bortezomib in autoimmune hemolytic anemia and beyond. Ther Adv Hematol 2021;12. 20406207211046428.

43. Crickx E, Audia S, Robbins A, et al. Daratumumab, an original approach for treating multi-refractory autoimmune cytopenia. Haematologica 2021. https://doi.org/10.3324/haematol.2021.279232.

44. Boccia R, Cooper N, Ghanima W, et al, FIT Clinical Trial Investigators. Fostamatinib is an effective second-line therapy in patients with immune thrombocytopenia. Br J Haematol 2020;190(6):933–93.

45. Serris A, Amoura Z, Canoui-Poitrine F, et al. Efficacy and safety of rituximab for systemic lupus erythematosus-associated immune cytopenias: a multicenter retrospective cohort study of 71 adults. Am J Hematol 2018;93:424–9.

46. Gobert D, Bussel JB, Cunningham-Rundles C, et al. Efficacy and safety of rituximab in common variable immunodeficiency-associated immune cytopenias: a retrospective multicentre study on 33 patients. Br J Haematol 2011;155(4): 498–508.

47. Guitton Z, Terriou L, Lega JC, et al. Risk of thrombosis with anti-phospholipid syndrome in systemic lupus erythematosus treated with thrombopoietin-receptor agonists. Rheumatology (Oxford) 2018;57(8):1432–8.

48. Rossignol J, Michallet AS, Oberic L, et al. Rituximab-cyclophosphamide-dexamethasone combination in the management of autoimmune cytopenias associated with chronic lymphocytic leukemia. Leukemia 2011;25(3):473–8.
49. Bride KL, Vincent T, Smith-Whitley K, et al. Sirolimus is effective in relapsed/refractory autoimmune cytopenias: results of a prospective multi-institutional trial. Blood 2016;127:17–28.